OXFORD MEDICAL PUBLICATIONS

Health Promotion
Models and Values

Health Promotion
Models and Values
Second Edition

R. S. DOWNIE
MA, B Phil, FRSE
Professor of Moral Philosophy
University of Glasgow

CAROL TANNAHILL
BA, MPH, PhD
Head of Health Promotion
Greater Glasgow Health Board

and

ANDREW TANNAHILL
MB, ChB, MSc, FFPHM, MHSM
General Manager
Health Education Board for Scotland

OXFORD
UNIVERSITY PRESS

OXFORD

UNIVERSITY PRESS

Great Clarendon Street, Oxford OX2 6DP

Oxford University Press is a department of the University of Oxford.
It furthers the University's objective of excellence in research, scholarship,
and education by publishing worldwide in

Oxford New York

Auckland Bangkok Buenos Aires Cape Town Chennai
Dar es Salaam Delhi Hong Kong Istanbul Karachi Kolkata
Kuala Lumpur Madrid Melbourne Mexico City Mumbai Nairobi
São Paulo Shanghai Singapore Taipei Tokyo Toronto
and an associated company in Berlin

Oxford is a registered trade mark of Oxford University Press
in the UK and in certain other countries

Published in the United States
by Oxford University Press Inc., New York

A catalogue record for this book is available from the British Library

Library of Congress Cataloging in Publication Data
(Data available)
ISBN 0 19 262591 8

Printed in Great Britain
on acid-free paper by
Biddles Ltd., Guildford and King's Lynn

Foreword

Kenneth Calman
Chief Medical Officer, Department of Health, London

The preservation and maintenance of health is of paramount importance to everyone. But what do we mean by health, and is it a social value, or a concept which relates solely to the individual? These questions have been part of our intellectual heritage for centuries, and are just as relevant today. In this book Professor Downie and Drs Tannahill bring together a philosophical and a practical approach to issues of health and health promotion in order to shed new light on the ways in which the public health can be improved.

An analysis of what determines health reveals that at least five factors interact to influence the health of an individual or population. These include *biological factors*, such as ageing and genetic changes; *lifestyle*, including behaviour; *environment*, which includes communicable diseases; *social and economic factors*; and *use of and access to health services*. With each of these factors there is a major role for health promotion in the improvement of the health of the population, emphasizing the definition of health arrived at in the book that 'health' is not an absolute concept, but something which can, and must, be constantly improved. Health targets therefore, such as lowering mortality rates, increasing uptake of immunization, changes in lifestyle etc., must not be seen as ends in themselves but as steps on the way to improving health and quality of life.

The book also emphasizes the fact that health has many dimensions, physical, social, psychological, and that it is not just a 'medical' issue but one which is relevant to all health care professionals, and the public at large. Part of this book therefore is concerned with the vocabulary of health promotion and how the words used by the public, the philosopher, the doctor, the educationalist, and many others, sometimes require clarification. Moreover, the same concept is sometimes called by a different name by different groups. Lifeskills, self-esteem, empowerment, and autonomy might be examples of such words.

A major part of this book is about evaluation, a key issue in health promotion. The approach taken is to identify the concepts involved and to provide an overview of this critical area. In a similar way the question of values in health and health promotion is tackled sensitively and in a practical way.

Scotland has a long and distinguished tradition of public health, which has always been concerned with the wider determinants of health including social and economic aspects, lifestyle, and the environment. This book, with which I am delighted to be associated, provides an important contribution to this tradition and a framework onto which health promotion projects can be built and evaluated.

There is an old Gaelic saying, 'Is e an oighreachd an t-slainte', which translated means 'Health is the inheritance'. This encapsulates much of the thought behind this book. Health and its promotion are to be seen not only in the short term but also require to be built into the consciousness of the public and professionals in order that change and improvement can be continually effected. Future generations may judge us by our response to issues relating to health.

Preface to the second edition

The 'health promotion movement' has gained ever more momentum in the 1990s, at international, national, and local levels. We have been pleased that our book has helped so many people to contribute to the impetus.

This updated and revised edition reflects developments in philosophy, policy, planning, and practice since the turn of the decade. We hope that it will enable us to continue to meet the need for a short textbook which both provides theoretical frameworks and demonstrates their practical value.

Glasgow   R.S.D.
December 1995   C.T.
                                                                    A.T.

Preface to the first edition

The overall philosophy of traditional health care is largely acceptable to the general public. The same cannot be said for health promotion, partly because it is a relatively new and unfamiliar field, but mainly due to the fact that it confronts many of our comfortable assumptions about health, medicine, lifestyle, and environment. Health promotion challenges us to see both ourselves and our society in a new light, and to alter radically the ways in which we perceive and pursue health. This book is aimed at helping people in a wide range of walks of life to rise to these challenges.

The multidisciplinary nature of health promotion is reflected in the collaboration of the three of us, from very different academic backgrounds, in furthering this aim. We have tried to integrate our various perspectives into a unified philosophy of health promotion, pulling together threads from medicine, education, social sciences, philosophy, and health promotion research and practice.

We hope that the book will be of interest and value to all those who have major contributions to make to health promotion and public health, including students and practitioners in the many branches of medicine and nursing, in health education/promotion, in environmental health, in education, and in social work, as well as politicians, community activists, and members of the public at large.

We are indebted to a number of friends and colleagues. We should like to thank especially Professor Kenneth Calman, who has taken time from his busy schedule as Chief Medical Officer for Scotland to write the Foreword. From his own clinical and teaching experience, and now from the perspective of a Government officer responsible for public health, he is well aware of the complexities of the issues we raise, and he is eminently well-suited to comment on them. We are most grateful to him.

Some of our thoughts on health, values, and justice are built on ideas first introduced in *Caring and Curing* (Downie and Telfer 1980), and we wish to thank Elizabeth Telfer for further discussing them. We also wish to acknowledge gratefully Graham Robertson, whose former close professional relationship with one of us (A.T.) helped with the sowing and germination of conceptual seeds.

Our handwriting and changes of mind have done nothing to enhance the well-being of our secretaries, Anne Valentine and Anne Southall, and we should like to thank them for the patience, diligence, and skill with which they tackled successive drafts of our text.

Glasgow   R.S.D.
April 1989   C.F.
                                                      A.T.

Contents

1 Introduction

The term 'health promotion' has come to refer to a movement which has gathered momentum over the past two decades. The movement is a radical one which challenges the medicalization of health, stresses its social and economic aspects, and portrays health as having a central place in a flourishing human life. The enthusiasm of those engaged in the movement has led to the development of many ideas on health and how it can be enhanced, but inevitably not all of these ideas are consistent, realistic, or well-articulated. This book is concerned with examining and developing out of these ideas workable models of health, its promotion, and its value base.

A whole host of individuals—professional and non-professional —and agencies—statutory and non-statutory—have major contributions to make to health promotion. This book is aimed at helping them towards a greater understanding of the principles of health promotion, an exploration of the underlying philosophy, and a fuller consideration of their actual and potential roles, in partnership with each other and with the communities they serve. We hope that the book will be of value in the preparation and development (formal and personal) of professionals in many fields, including medicine, nursing, other health professions, social work, school and community education, and community development.

The material is presented in two parts. Part 1 embraces key principles of health promotion and offers models for definition, planning, and action. It builds on a broad theoretical base derived from behavioural and educational sciences, epidemiology and clinical practice, and philosophy. This part of the book, although essentially theoretical, is firmly orientated towards practicality, and indeed concludes with a series of examples of principles in practice. To a large extent it represents a distillation of the discussions which constitute Part 2 of the book. The order is intentional: the reader has, through Part 1, easy and immediate access to frameworks for action, and this is backed up by the more detailed account and debate in Part 2.

The central concept of health promotion, and the launching pad of many of its most exciting ideas, is health itself. Accordingly, we begin with an examination of the concept of health, taking as our initial text the much quoted and widely criticized World Health Organization (WHO) definition of health:

Health is a state of complete physical, mental and social well-being, and not merely the absence of disease or infirmity.

This definition makes several important points for our purposes.

First of all, it involves a distinction between health negatively defined—as the absence of ill-health—and health as a positive state—seen as the presence of well-being. Developing this distinction, we assign a substantial amount of our next chapter to the delineation of the negative and positive dimensions of health, and their complex interrelationships. We broaden out from the WHO conception of positive health to include fitness in addition to well-being.

Secondly, the WHO definition includes mental and social as well as physical aspects of health. We acknowledge the importance of these neglected areas, giving some attention to the mental aspects in Chapter 2, and a much larger treatment to the social in Part 2. The unified and enlarged concept of health we argue to be rooted in, and an expression of, the more general idea of the good or flourishing life for human beings. We elaborate this position in our account of fundamental human values in Part 2.

Some of the many uncertainties generated by the health promotion movement concern its relationship to longer established interests of health professionals—health education and public health. Two chapters are therefore given over to advancing models of health education and health promotion, concluding with a brief consideration of their relation to public health. Out of this discussion emerges our recommended definition of health promotion:

Health promotion comprises efforts to enhance positive health and reduce the risk of ill-health, through the overlapping spheres of health education, prevention, and health protection.

Some have seen in health promotion ways of cutting costs in traditional health care. But this raises many questions. How do we know whether a health promotion initiative has been effective? Is it just a matter of saving money? Is it mainly to do with increasing people's knowledge of health and its determinants? In a chapter on evaluation we try to show that these and related questions are more complex than they at first seem. In the end, we conclude that health promotion is justifiable on its aims alone, rather than depending on economic arguments.

In dealing with values we note in several contexts that they can be described in different ways, and that new terminology is sometimes introduced for ideas which are familiar in traditional terminology. This is inevitable, in that health promotion is an eclectic discipline and its practitioners come to it from a variety of backgrounds with their own terminologies. For example, health promotion stresses the importance of acquiring 'lifeskills'; but this is just new nomenclature for what, in the philosophy of education, has been called 'self-development'. Again, 'self-esteem' has taken the place of the more traditional 'self-respect'.

We ask our readers to consider how far the concepts of their own disciplines, or of ordinary vocabulary, can be exchanged with or translated into the concepts of health promotion. For instance, medical, nursing, social work, and other health care professionals will be familiar with the concept of 'autonomy' (itself drawn from eighteenth-century philosophy). The health promotion movement stresses the importance of what it calls 'empowerment'. But the concept of empowerment simply serves to bring out the fact that many people, whether because of poor health, inadequate housing, unemployment, or low self-esteem, do not have autonomy, or the ability adequately to make choices and determine their own lives. People must therefore be enabled and encouraged to develop autonomy—they must, in a word, be 'empowered'.

One of the key concepts for health promotion is that of an attitude. The concept of an attitude is central because it brings together beliefs, emotions, and behaviour. We therefore devote a chapter to analysing what it means to hold an attitude, and to suggesting ways in which attitudes can be changed; for the bringing about of changes in attitudes, and in associated behaviour, is one of the objectives of health promotion.

It is, among other things, because it attempts to bring about changes in attitudes and behaviour that health promotion inevitably generates objections. Many of these objections contain points of substance, and we have therefore devoted a chapter in this second edition to discussing them. Our discussion of the objections, like much else in the book, rests on a firm value-base.

It is therefore necessary to discuss valuing and values. We suggest that the realization of certain values is necessary for the flourishing of human society and human personality. Health itself is a central concept here, for it is one of the values which is not only an essential *means to* human flourishing, but is itself an *expression of* human flourishing. Health is like education in that it is both an 'enabling' good—good for what it brings—and also good in itself, or worthwhile for its own sake.

The majority of writings on health promotion acknowledge the importance of values and the ethical problems of health promotion, but they assign only a small place to the detailed analysis of values and valuing. We try to supplement these writings by bringing out the modifications which health promotion is committed to making in our liberal-democratic tradition—away from an individualistic interpretation of that tradition and back to one based on citizenship.

In view of its commitment to change in individual and social values, health promotion is a politically sensitive activity. For example, it cannot be denied that important determinants of health are the material and social environments. Poor housing, poor education, polluted atmosphere, and unemployment are all factors affecting health, and are all factors with a high political profile. It is therefore impossible to discuss health promotion without being seen as adopting a political stance. We stress that the principles of health promotion will inevitably have political implications, but that it is important to build practice and arguments for change on the solid foundations of these basic principles, rather than resorting to the shorthand vocabulary of politics.

Health care professionals of all kinds, including those involved in health education and health promotion, tend to be practical people who are to an extent suspicious of theory. There is sometimes a contrast implied in health promotion literature between theory, depicted as 'airy-fairy', and practice, depicted as 'down-to-earth'. But we do not necessarily know where we are going or what we are doing just because we claim to be 'down-to-earth'. There is a well-known saying which warns us against not being able to see the wood for the trees! To know where we are going, to have a clear view of the wood, it can be helpful to make an occasional aerial survey. In other words, we must have a good grasp of a philosophy of health promotion, its principles and justification, or we shall be lost in a morass of empirical detail and tips for day-to-day business. Our book is an attempt to state this philosophy explicitly.

There are other reasons for having a clear philosophy of health promotion. The general public and the traditional health care professions can be sceptical of the activities of health promotion, suggesting that anything worthwhile in the movement is done by traditional medicine anyway, and that the rest is just gratuitous interference with lifestyle. It is thus important for those involved with health promotion to be clear on their answers to the questions: 'What is health promotion *for*?'; 'What is distinctive about it?'; and 'Why is it worthwhile?' We therefore hope that our book will provide:

(1) a *a bird's eye view of the nature* of health promotion;

(2) an account of its *links* with related health care activities;

(3) a *justification* for it and what it is attempting to do;

(4) an *underlying support* or *value base* for its practical activities.

In the film *Educating Rita*, Rita, having begun her education, goes back to the pub with her parents and listens to the singing. She is dissatisfied with it and says: 'There must be better tunes'. Health promotion seems to us to be committed to the belief that indeed there are better tunes—better and worse lifestyles. This is not to say that there is only one good way to live, but unless we are convinced that some lifestyles are better than others for helping human nature to flourish we can see no point in health promotion.

Part 1 Models

2 Health

The growth of interest and activity in health promotion in recent times has been accompanied by many attempts to delineate health itself. This is understandable: it may be reasonably argued that, just as a history or chemistry teacher needs to know his or her subject in order to teach it, so must a 'health promoter' have a clear idea of what it is that is to be promoted.

Attempts at delineating health have been directed along two lines: the pursuit of a neat definition, and the description of a number of 'models' of health. Neither set of efforts has been entirely successful. In the first place, the simple intuitive notions which we all have about our own (and others') health have proved not to be readily translatable into a brief but adequate definition. Secondly, models—'biomedical', 'social', 'welfare', and the like—have been falsely presented as distinct aspects or views of health in watertight compartments, with consequent neglect of how the various components are integrated.

In this chapter, we explore the meaning of health and construct a model which seeks to pull together the many and varied strands that together constitute health. This enables us to identify an overall goal for health promotion.

2.1 Defining health

The most commonly quoted definition of health, as noted in our introductory chapter, is that presented in the Constitution of the World Health Organization (WHO 1946):

Health is a state of complete physical, mental and social well-being, and not merely the absence of disease or infirmity.

This definition has been widely criticized. However, as we shall show, there are merits along with the shortcomings. In the first instance we shall concentrate on only one aspect of the definition, namely the distinction between negative and positive aspects of health.

The former is negative in two respects: health is viewed (in a negative sense) as involving the *absence* of disease or infirmity (themselves *negative* in connotation). Similarly, the latter is positive in two ways: health is seen (positively) as entailing the *presence* of a (*positive*) quality—well-being.

No matter how often the WHO definition or similar constructs are cited by health professionals (among others), it is true to say that in practice the positive aspect of health tends to be neglected. It is a well-worn but nonetheless true cliché that we have a National *Sickness* Service rather than a National Health Service. Even with the rise of health promotion, attention has been skewed towards the prevention of ill-health as opposed to the promotion of the positive dimension.

2.2 Negative health

The familiar, and currently dominant, negative dimension of health—which we shall refer to as *ill-health*—is not as straightforward as may be assumed. In speaking about ill-health, one might be referring to disease, injury, illness, disability, or handicap, singly or in various combinations and experienced over a long or a short period of time.

Disease and illness are not synonymous. Someone may feel, and be seen to be, ill as a result of a diagnosed disease. Someone else, on the other hand, may have a disease without any illness manifestation, for example a skin condition presenting only as a rash, or even a presymptomatic cancer. Equally, another person may feel or look ill in the absence of a disease or injury: he or she may be situationally depressed, or have taken an overdose, or simply have a hangover. Clearly, to describe ill-health in terms either of disease or of illness would be incomplete without mention of the other; we shall therefore have to give an account of ill-health in terms of both notions. Let us explore their meaning and relationship further.

2.2.1 Disease and illness as disorders

Illness is a less technical notion than disease. Any lay person, including the sufferer, can know that someone is ill without

knowing whether or not he or she has a disease, let alone what
disease it is. At least this is true of physical illness; mental illness,
as we shall see, may be more difficult. Taking physical illness only
for the time being, let us consider what makes someone say that
he or she (or another person) is ill. Relevant factors are what many
would call overall upsets of the system: for example, not wanting
to eat, feeling and being weak, feeling abnormally hot or cold, or
having a weak pulse. People who are ill will often have headaches
or rashes or itches, but these isolated phenomena would not in
themselves constitute being ill. Thus someone can say: 'When I
had German measles I came out in a splendid rash but I wasn't ill
at all', meaning that he or she was not (or not very) feverish, ate
normally, felt strong, etc. Again, people who have a stye or boil
are not ill simply thereby, although if they get a fever as a result
of this kind of infection, they are then said to be ill.

So far we have made no distinction between *being* ill and *feeling*
ill. The sense of this distinction is far from clear. One distinction
might be between the symptoms of which only the sufferer is
aware—aches and pains, feelings of faintness or nausea—and the
signs which can be detected by others, such as raised temperature
or quickened pulse. If a patient reports a series of untoward
feelings but the doctor can 'find nothing' he or she might say,
'You aren't really ill.' Similarly, persons with German measles
who have a rash but feel fine, instead of saying 'I'm not ill' might
equally well say 'I don't *feel* ill', implying that since they have
German measles they *are* in fact ill.

But this distinction between the objective conditions and the
subjective ones is not an exhaustive account of the difference
between being ill and feeling ill. For, if people go on reporting
headaches, giddiness, and so on of sufficient severity, and we
believe them, we might well say not just that they *feel* ill, but
that they *are* ill with some as yet mysterious condition. Of course,
many a doctor in such a case may say (or at any rate think):
'You're not really ill, it's just your nerves.' But then the same
view could be expressed, perhaps more charitably, by saying 'It's
your nerves which are making you ill.' The distinction between
being and feeling ill, then, is sometimes between the objective and
the subjective, sometimes between the temporary and persistent,
and sometimes between the mental and the physical.

Disease is a more technical notion than illness, as we said earlier.
A person who has a disease suffers from some medically defined

condition which is identifiable as similar to that suffered from by some others.

A crucial notion in both illness and disease is that of *upset* or *disorder*. We can partly understand this if we think of the human body as a machine, in which various processes (such as digestion and excretion, maintenance of a certain temperature, inhaling of oxygen) necessary to its maintenance and smooth working are carried out, and through which the person whose body it is carries out his or her actions. On this model an upset or disorder would be some failure in the system which prevented the machine working properly, and what was wrong or bad about it would be precisely this interference with the machine's normal working.

2.2.2 Disease and illness as unwanted states

The above mechanistic model of ill-health is only partly satisfactory. For one thing, it does not accommodate pain and other subjective symptoms, such as nausea, feeling faint, etc. It might be retorted that this is in the nature of the case, since pain and other feelings are essentially inward and non-mechanistic. In any case, it might be said, they are indicators of the disorder rather than parts of it and so their analogue in mechanical terms would be with the untoward sounds with which motorists become obsessed. But this will not quite do either. There can be pain with no apparent organic cause, and in a case like this we would not say: 'Since the mechanism is working normally that's all that matters.' The pain itself constitutes a disorder which must be put right. No doubt if severe it will psychologically interfere with the sufferer's activities, but even where it does not, the presence of pain is still in itself a matter for medical attention, and a person in pain, even from no apparent cause, is regarded as ill or at any rate not well.

So far, then, we have two kinds of phenomena that constitute ill-health: what may be termed mechanical failure, and some other discomfort. Is there any way of linking these two factors? One possible line which suggests itself is that both pain and malfunction are *unpleasant* things for those who have them. This assertion would, of course, need a little qualification. Some pain, in some circumstances, can be pleasant, and illness can be positively welcome—if for example it gets one out of the Army. But in general terms pain is unpleasant, and, in general, being incapacitated prevents people from doing whatever they want to do—at least as regards normal plans and projects. Can we then say that the disorder which characterizes illness and disease, and which takes the form both of discomfort and of mechanical failure, is to be described as a (physical) condition which is in general unpleasant or prevents people from doing what they want?

2.2.3 Disease and illness as abnormal states

This will not do, for there are examples of such conditions which are clearly not illnesses, for instance the weakness and loss of faculties that accompany ageing. These are not regarded as illnesses because they are 'natural' or 'normal'. In other words, everyone goes through something of the kind, or at any rate suffers some out of a range of unpleasant changes. There is therefore an idea of the *normal* against which certain kinds of change are judged to be illnesses, others not. In a similar way, the pains of childbirth, arising as they do from a natural process, are regarded as normal, rather as aching muscles after strenuous or unaccustomed exercise are regarded as normal.

We can say, then, that a condition is to be regarded as a disorder, and not merely as unpleasant, by reference to a conception of a normal state for human beings. The aspect of abnormality is indeed uppermost in some cases of disease. As we said earlier, minor skin diseases may not make a person ill in any way or cause any discomfort, and what makes them *diseases* is that they constitute abnormal conditions of the skin. Of course, they are as a rule undesirable to their possessor, because they are unsightly, but the verdict of unsightliness is largely dependent on the judgement of abnormality.

2.2.4 Disabilities, deformities, and unwanted states

At this point it may well be objected that to distinguish normal from abnormal changes and call only the latter illnesses and diseases is totally artificial, as doctors and others are also concerned with trying to arrest normal changes if they are undesirable; for example, to lessen the effects of ageing with appropriate diet and exercise, or hormone therapy. It is important to note, however, that if young children have stiff joints we might say there is something wrong with them, whereas if old people have stiff joints we might say that they are not as agile as they were. There is a difference not only in how the two situations are described, but also in how they are dealt with. No doubt doctors do try to alleviate such concomitants of old age but, if the two disabilities were equal, there would be much more doubt about spending a lot of effort on such activity than there would be in the case of the child because there is an idea that older people 'shouldn't expect' to be as mobile as they were.

A parallel situation occurs with regard to deformity and less obvious cosmetic problems. Certainly, doctors do regard it as part of their business to correct abnormalities of appearance (with plastic surgery) if they are extreme, but if they are mild they do not seem to make the automatic claim for aid that a deformity such as harelip does. Similarly, they will regard it as their business to alleviate the pains of childbirth if required to do so, but there is no expectation that all trace of discomfort will be relieved. In our conception of disease and illness, then, there is a built-in implication of some normal condition of the human body by reference to which these things are aberrations.

2.2.5 Disease and illness as 'law-like'

We have said that deformity is analogous to illness in being a disorder which medicine is concerned to treat—or better still, of course, to prevent. But it should be noticed that deformity, unlike some illness and disease, is not as such incompatible with good health. Of course, there are some deformities, such as 'holes in the heart', which produce mechanical failures, and a sufferer from these is said to be in poor health. But a child who is born deaf is not merely by dint of this defect called unhealthy. It is true that a person who is severely handicapped in this way might hesitate before stating on a form that he or she is in good health, but broadly speaking these handicaps, severe though they are, are somehow not thought of as impairing *health*. This is difficult to understand in terms of our account so far, which depicts ill-health as uncomfortable or frustrating abnormalities of a system.

The explanation seems to be that illness and disease are seen as things which essentially progress or change in a law-like manner, which have a life of their own. In such cases one can always sensibly ask whether the sufferer is getting better or worse. Being ill is essentially an unstable situation. The deaf child, by contrast, is fixed in disability, and so not regarded as unhealthy because there is nothing untoward going on in him or her. But the fact, if it is one, that the deformed person is not regarded as unhealthy does not mean that doctors or others have no concern with trying to prevent such cases or to alleviate their lot—with false limbs, plastic surgery, etc. What it means, rather, is that health, in the negative sense, is too narrow to be regarded as the goal of health care. What we need instead is some notion of positive health or physical 'wholeness' which includes not only what is implied by the absence of ill-health but additional elements. We shall pick up on this notion in due course.

2.2.6 Injury

It should be noted that some of the points which apply to deformity apply also to *injury*. Sometimes people who have been badly injured are described as ill, and when this is so they are suffering from the same kinds of incapacity that attend other illness—weakness, faintness, unconsciousness, etc. But if the lack of capacity is simply the essential result of the injury, then the sufferer might in one sense be in good health. A skier who has broken a leg cannot walk, but may be in glowing health. The doctor's task here may again be described as the restoration not of health but of wholeness. But injury is in one respect more like illness than deformity: it can progress in that it can heal.

We can summarize this account of physical ill-health by saying that it can occur in episodes or over long periods, that it can manifest itself in illness, disease, deformity, or injury, and that these overlapping concepts can be linked if they are seen on the model of *abnormal, unwanted,* or *incapacitating* states of a biological system.

2.2.7 Mental and social ill-health

So far we have concentrated on *physical* ill-health, as still often happens in discussions of health and in health service planning and practice. The situation becomes even more complex when we remind ourselves of the existence of the very important mental and social facets. Important concepts touched on above as part of physical ill-health—disease, injury, illness, disability, and handicap—may be applied, albeit with varying readiness, to both of these additional elements of health.

We summarized our views of physical ill-health by saying that it consists of the presence of physically *abnormal conditions* (such as diseases or deformities) and/or *unwanted conditions* (such as skin rashes) and/or *incapacitating conditions* (such as injuries to limbs). Let us try to carry these ideas over to the spheres of the mental and social. Take first abnormality.

The idea of abnormal or sick states of mind is much less obvious and a source of much more disagreement than that of abnormal bodily states. The reason for this is that in the case of the body the 'abnormal' is specified in terms of an objective biological norm, whereas in the case of the mind the norm is a culturally relative, social, or statistical norm. Moreover, the further suggestion that anyone who has an abnormal state of mind is mentally ill is at the beginning of a path which leads to the conclusion that 'immorality', or even the non-conformity of minority social groups, as examples of 'deviance', are forms of mental illness. To construe any 'deviant' behaviour as being necessarily the product of 'sick' or 'abnormal' desires and therefore a sign of mental illness is to give a spurious air of objectivity to what is largely culture-relative, and it may also be to deny responsibility for action to those regarded as social wrong-doers. It is down this road that we encounter the Soviet psychiatrists who used to treat as mentally ill those who criticized the regime.

Confusion over the idea of abnormal states of mind is due to the fact that three different concepts are being run together—sick desires, minority desires, and immoral or illegal desires. It is not easy to draw satisfying distinctions between these concepts, but we might say that a 'sick' desire is one which people cannot make sense of in terms of their own experience, and which is destructive of human personality. A minority or eccentric desire is one which (statistically) is not common, but it may or may not be 'sick', 'immoral', or 'illegal'—for example, a desire to collect old typewriters. An immoral or illegal desire is harmful to the person concerned or to society generally, but it may or may not be sick and it may or may not be minority. For example, a desire to steal one's neighbour's property is (perhaps) a minority desire, it is immoral (and illegal if implemented), but it is not sick. But a desire to collect nail clippings from corpses is sick, because it bears no relation to any of the reasons for which people collect things, and it is obviously a minority desire; but it is not as such immoral since it causes no harm. This way of drawing the line between the three classes of desire, all called 'abnormal', is only rough and ready, but scientific precision cannot be expected. Nevertheless, the distinctions are important.

The second idea of mental illness, as an unwanted state, is also difficult. In the case of physical illness it is the sufferers themselves who do not want the condition in which they find themselves. But in the case of mental illness what is wrong, sometimes at least, is that sufferers are content with the state they are in. Of course, the fact that someone has sick desires in itself gives no warrant for interfering with him or her. The psychopath, on the other hand, is harming others—other people suffer from the state more directly than he or she—and one thing wrong with the psychopath is precisely that he or she is not disturbed by the sick wants and does not request that they be treated. Hence, whereas some of those who are mentally ill may want to be rid of their states, this is by no means characteristic and there are therefore uncertainties in the carry-over of the idea of unwanted states from physical to mental ill-health.

To try to avoid the difficulties in the idea of unwanted states we can turn to the third strand in the concept of ill-health—that of loss of capacity. According to this account, just as physical disease means that the body cannot fulfil its function, so mental disease means that people cannot do what they are normally able to do in the mental sphere—reason, understand their world, or exercise their will. On this account, typical cases of mental illness are obsessive-compulsive neurosis (showing itself, for example, in repetitive actions which the patient cannot help doing), or incapacitating depression. But it would follow that psychopathy, showing itself not in loss of capacity but in frightful behaviour which the agent wilfully carries out, is not a mental illness at all. That conclusion is counter-intuitive, and hence we need all three accounts of mental ill-health, as with physical ill-health—in terms of abnormal states, unwanted states, and incapaciting states.

2.2.8 Summary

The physical, mental, and social *facets* of ill-health are inextricably interlinked: serious or troublesome physical illness, for example, may lead to mental ill-health (a depressive or anxiety state, perhaps) or social impairment; likewise mental illness may result in physical ill-health (such as injury arising from failed suicide) or social handicap. Similarly, physical, mental, and social *factors*—determinants of ill-health—may respectively damage other aspects of health: for instance, low socio-economic status is associated with a wide range of physical and mental health problems.

Given the complexity of ill-health—with its physical, mental, and social facets and determinants, and its subjective and objective aspects—a person's level of ill-health is clearly far less straightforward to assess fully than is perhaps implied from the day-to-day work of doctors and other health professionals.

2.3 Well-being

We shall now move on to consider the positive dimension of health as embraced by the WHO definition—well-being. Let us begin by attempting to provide an analysis of a complex concept.

We shall look first at *feelings* of well-being. 'Well-being' sometimes means no more than people's subjective estimations of mood or level of happiness on a given occasion. In this sense, they themselves are the only authority on their well-being, and there is no implication as to how they have come to be in that state or how long it will last. If they are 'feeling great' then they have a high degree of subjective well-being whether that state will last minutes or a lifetime, whether it is brought about by being in love, going for a swim, good weather, or alcohol.

Subjective well-being, however, may be spurious. It may arise from influences which are overall detrimental to an individual's functioning or flourishing, and/or to society. In other words, as with ill-health, we must look to a more objective assessment of well-being. In doing so it is important to pay attention to the *origins* of feelings of well-being.

To take a crude example, the notion of the enhancement of well-being as a pre-eminent goal of health promotion has been questioned by some who would suggest that this goal could be achieved by the mass administration of heroin to the population. One could not reasonably argue that narcotic-induced euphoria constitutes a state of positive health. Similarly, it would be difficult to make a case for viewing an acute schizophrenic state with mood elevation and a blissful lack of insight as one of positive health. Subjective well-being, then, must stand up to some sort of outside scrutiny if we are to consider it to be a true state of well-being—reflecting positive health. As part of this scrutiny we must look critically at the *basis* of feelings of well-being. We argue that *true* well-being involves and reflects a quality which we shall refer to as *empowerment*, and which we examine below.

This concept of true well-being is much more structured than that of subjective well-being, and contains essential reference to some conception of the 'good life' for a human being. A great deal of wisdom has been accumulated over the centuries about the kinds of activities which make for a flourishing human life. Important here will be some conception of having a measure of control over one's life, of being able to choose what one wants to do or be, and of being able to develop one's talents. This strand in the idea of well-being has a social and political side to it as well. Experience teaches that, on the whole, most people have a much more lasting and deeper level of well-being (or happiness) if they have friends, if they have some confidence that their material needs are going to be satisfied, if they are not going to be put in prison in an arbitrary way, and so on. We shall say much more about this strand to well-being in Chapters 9–11, where we shall connect it with the more traditional concept of autonomy and the newer expression of autonomy in the idea of empowerment.

Subjective (or hedonistic) well-being, then, can exist with or without true ('good life') well-being. It *can* be brought about by acquiring lifeskills and achieving autonomy or empowerment. This point is of the first importance for health promotion and indeed for health care more generally. Let us take an example. Imagine a single parent who consults her general practitioner (GP) because she feels depressed. The temptation for the GP may well be to prescribe an anxiolytic drug which will make the patient feel better about herself and her situation. In other words, the GP can induce a state of subjective well-being. The disadvantage of this approach is that the well-being depends on the continuing use of the drug. On the other hand, the approach of a health educationist might be to encourage the single parent to be in touch with others in similar situations and to get all the financial and other support to which she is legally entitled. In other words, the second approach is directed towards the acquisition or development of lifeskills and autonomy, or empowerment.

This second approach to the promotion of well-being is slower, but it is the only one which in the long term will achieve a lasting, true well-being. To say this is not, of course, to suggest that there may not be contexts for short-term remedies, or to underestimate the problems in the second method. We shall discuss in more detail the concepts of the objectivist, 'good life' approach to well-being in later chapters (see especially Chapter 9). In the meantime it is sufficient to note that the biomedical approach to health tends to involve the subjective sense of well-being since it can be drug-induced, whereas the health promotion approach, with its stress on 'being all you can be', must assume the second, 'good life' sense.

2.4 Linking well-being and ill-health

Let us now turn to look at the connection between well-being and ill-health. Attempts to relate the two concepts or similar ideas have generally taken the form of a continuum (Catford 1983), with extremes of well-being and ill-health at the positive and negative ends, respectively (Fig. 2.1).

Ill-health ←   → Well-being
(−)   0   (+)

Fig. 2.1 Health as a continuum.

Even leaving aside objections (religious and otherwise) to the tendency to present death as the ultimate in ill-health rather than an ultimate consequence of it, this sort of schema is unsatisfactory. It is possible to feel full of well-being in the presence of serious or even life-threatening disease; equally one may be free of illness, with the benefit of medical evidence, without enjoying a feeling of well-being. It thus makes more sense to present well-being and ill-health as two axes at right angles to, and crossing, each other (Fig. 2.2). Since ill-health is a negative entity, the horizontal axis is presented, somewhat unusually, as having 'high' to the left and 'low' to the right. This has the effect of preserving the mathematical convention of positive x and y co-ordinates in the right upper quadrant, making for easier conceptualization.

We shall now consider four individuals (numbered 1 to 4) plotted on Fig. 2.2 according to characteristics of (true) well-being and ill-health at a given point in time.

Fig. 2.2 The relationship between well-being and ill-health.

1. This individual is free of ill-health, and this is matched by a high level of well-being. This is clearly a highly desirable state.
2. This person has a high level of ill-health and a correspondingly low level of well-being. He or she may, for example, have terminal cancer, be in a great deal of pain, and feel desolate.
3. The third individual does not feel ill, and has no other evidence of ill-health, but for some reason this state is accompanied by a low level of well-being. He or she may, for instance, feel too socially unskilled or physically unfit to enjoy a 'clean bill of health'.
4. This person is experiencing a high level of well-being despite a high level of ill-health. Such people may feel in peak physical condition, unaware of an advanced malignancy, or may be terminally ill but well-adjusted to their fate, at peace with themselves and the world.

The reader may have noticed the physical, mental, and social facets of well-being alluded to above, consistent with the WHO view of health. As is the case with negative health, levels of well-being according to the three sets of criteria may be similar or different at any time. Also, like ill-health, aspects of well-being may be short-lived (especially in the case of purely subjective well-being) or longer term.

2.5 Fitness

Another quality commonly arises in discussion of *positive health*, namely *fitness*. Consideration of this characteristically focuses on *physical* attributes, commonly 'the Four S's': Strength, Stamina, Suppleness, and Skills. We shall therefore start on familiar territory, by considering physical fitness as an element of positive health.

Criteria for assessing physical fitness form a spectrum in which we can distinguish three main points. At one end of this spectrum, fitness is viewed simply as the ability to execute ordinary, everyday tasks without undue physical discomfort (such as muscle aches). It is assessed in relation to targets arising from a person's normal daily life, and according to the presence, absence, or degree of physical consequences of carrying out routine activities. Individuals have their own personal indicators of physical fitness, integral to their life situation—such as being able to run for a bus, or carry a child or a load of bricks. As long as people manage to attain their own targets with regard to their particular set of indicators, they may regard themselves as fit, according to this minimalist view of physical fitness. Personal indicators and targets will, naturally, vary throughout someone's life, in relation to age, disability, etc.

Moving along the spectrum of functioning to a second points, we may adopt a more refined view of physical fitness by seeing it in terms of suitability to perform highly specialized roles or tasks. For example, someone may be considered, on the basis of certain criteria, to be fit to be a dancer in a particular *corps de ballet*, or a player in a given football team. Particular aspects of physical fitness need to be developed to a given degree for a special purpose. As with the minimalist view, fitness is seen as a means to an end.

At the opposite end of the spectrum from the minimalist view we have a third idea, that of maximizing the efficiency and effectiveness of the body as a machine: developing the capacity of the heart as a pump, of the lungs as gas exchangers, and of body muscles as sources of power. Efforts to maximize physical fitness may be a means to an end: training may be aimed at one's capabilities in a specific role (such as sprinting or dancing), and fitness will then be gauged according to performance in that role. This is not always the case, however. People may seek to develop physical fitness as an end in itself: tests of fitness may become relegated to a series of gymnasium tests and visual assessment of muscle bulk; pursuit of fitness may become an obsession, divorced from the basic requirements for a balanced and fruitful life.

It is easy to see that physical fitness will often be accompanied by feelings of well-being. Indeed, true physical fitness (as distinct from spurious feelings which could not stand up to some sort of test) might reasonably be seen as the physical counterpart of the essentially mental and social qualities of empowerment referred to in Section 2.3. Furthermore, one might even argue that the concept of a functional spectrum of physical fitness—from *minimalist* through *specialist* to *maximalist*—is also applicable to mental and social considerations. Such explorations lead us rapidly into murky waters, however, and so we shall move on without further discussion to a relatively simple, but nonetheless useful, delineation of positive health.

2.6 Positive health

We see positive health as comprising true well-being (with its roots in empowerment, and of considerable value to the individual and society) together with the related notion of fitness, and as having physical, mental, and social ingredients. We shall go no further towards attempting to tease out these threads.

We consider that a state of positive health involves high levels of both components, true well-being and fitness. Moreover, such a state entails an appropriate *balance* of the physical, mental, and social ingredients: over-concentration on one may be to the detriment of either or both of the others. For example, an extreme commitment to physical training may interfere with the development or maintenance of mental or social skills, and may militate against mental and social well-being.

2.7 A model of health

We shall now examine how a model of health may be synthesized from the complex and interrelated ingredients which we have identified in this chapter, with a view to elucidating an overall goal for health promotion.

First we shall return to the WHO definition of health. We whole-
heartedly approve of the way in which this definition alerts one to
the inextricably interlinked physical, mental, and social facets of
health, and to its positive and negative dimensions. However, we
have drawn attention to the inadequacy of regarding *all* well-being
as indicative of positive health (recall the distinction between
spurious and true well-being). Furthermore, we have raised the
concept of fitness as part of positive health. Moreover, we join with
others before us in criticizing the Utopian nature of the construct in
describing a 'complete state'. Finally, we suggest that the definition
is misleading in implying that health is an *absolute* concept. Rather,
we see health as *relative*: health promotion must help people to *better* health rather than seeking to attain a specified *level* of health.

The model shown as Fig. 2.3 is an attempt to summarize the
elements of health and their interrelationships.

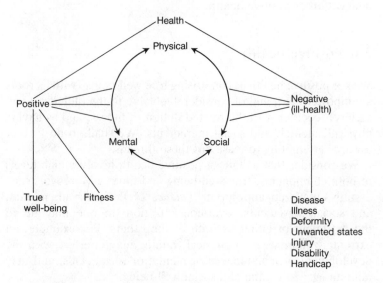

Fig. 2.3 A model of health.

Both positive and negative health are to be seen as having
interconnected physical, mental, and social elements. The representation of these facets as bridges between positive and negative
reminds us that levels of positive health and ill-health in relation to
one particular facet often go hand in hand; physical illness may well
be accompanied by a low level of physical well-being or fitness, for

instance. We should, however, remember from the earlier account that well-being is not always inversely related to ill-health; neither is fitness invariably thus related to ill-health—someone may have cancer but be fit, for example. Indeed, we can represent the relationship between positive health—comprising true well-being and fitness—and ill-health by substituting 'positive health' for 'well-being' in Fig. 2.2.

Health has to be seen as the sum or product of all its components, and, if we bear in mind the complexity of the many points we have made in this chapter, we see that the *precise* quantification of an individual's health, let alone a population's, is impossible. When we speak of 'improving health' (or, in modern parlance, 'improving health status'), we must be referring to increasing the overall 'quantity' of health, by enhancing positive health, reducing negative health, or both. It may clearly be very difficult to judge whether 'health gain', at the level of the individual or on a population scale, has indeed taken place as a result of intervention, given the unpredictable relationship between positive and negative health, and the interconnections between physical, mental, and social facets. The final decision is likely to be based on value judgements—on whether the positive dimension is given precedence over the negative, on the relative importance attached to physical, mental, and social criteria, and so on. Self-perceived health may thus differ significantly from others-perceived, not just because of the presence of 'untestable' subjective elements of health as described earlier, but also as a result of differing value systems. The issue of measuring health is discussed more fully in Chapter 5.

2.8 The goal of health promotion

The lack of a clear-cut, predictable association between negative and positive health has implications for the goal of health promotion. Health promotion must seek to prevent ill-health in such a way as simultaneously to enhance positive health: blinkered attention to prevention might result in behaviour geared so much to risk avoidance that positive health—both well-being and fitness—would suffer. Health promotion must also attempt to develop positive health with an eye on prevention: for example, encouragement to take physical exercise, through cycling or running, perhaps, should take into account the risks of injury, and should build in appropriate safety measures.

The *overall goal* of health promotion may be summed up as *the balanced enhancement of physical, mental, and social facets of positive health, coupled with the prevention of physical, mental, and social ill-health*.

The reader should not be discouraged from developing his or her role in health promotion as a result of the breadth of scope of this goal. While we should certainly encourage everyone to consider carefully the full range of his or her potential contributions, we freely admit that the individual is unlikely to be in a position to contribute greatly towards all the various components of the goal. Indeed, the pressing message is that a great many individuals and agencies have parts to play in health promotion, and should work together towards achieving its overall goal.

2.9 Conclusions

1. The WHO definition of health distinguishes a positive and a negative dimension to health.
2. Negative health, or ill-health, has a subjective component expressed in the concepts of illness and discomfort, and an objective component expressed in concepts of disease, injury, handicap, or deformity. These strands are linked via the idea of abnormal, unwanted, or incapacitating states of a biological system, which in turn presupposes the idea of a good or flourishing human life.
3. These ideas can be carried over to the spheres of the mental and social.
4. Positive health has two components: well-being and fitness.
5. Well-being can be purely subjective, but to be a component of positive health it must arise from and reflect a process of empowerment, which may be enhanced through the development of lifeskills.
6. Fitness can be seen on a spectrum from minimalist through functionalist to maximalist.
7. The overall goal of health promotion is the balanced enhancement of physical, mental, and social positive health, coupled with the prevention of physical, mental, and social ill-health.
8. A great many individuals and agencies may work together towards this goal.

3 Health education

Health promotion is rooted in the narrower, more established field of health education. The widespread and burgeoning interest in health promotion must take due account of the lessons to be learnt from health education: health promotion will otherwise transpire to be a mere veneer, an inadequate usurper of health education rather than a more powerful force for change. Consequently, this chapter examines the evolution and principles of health education, as a prelude to detailed consideration of health promotion (Chapter 4).

People have firm, and varied, views regarding the nature of health education. Interpretations are influenced by professional background and experience and, among other factors, by perceptions of the meanings of the component words, 'health' and 'education'. Too often health education is perceived by powerful individuals and groups (such as politicians, health service managers, and doctors) as being essentially a simple matter of telling people what they ought to do to be healthy. Dangerous oversimplifications of this sort among key potential health educators have gone hand in hand with a tendency for health education to be treated as an 'instant expert' subject, with preconceptions and intuition in place of experience and rigour. This chapter is aimed primarily at helping the vast and varied legions of health educators to a common understanding of the principles and scope of health education.

3.1 Definitions

Many definitions of health education have been offered in recent years. We shall consider only two.

Smith's (1979) definition suggests that we all receive 'health education' of various sorts as we simply go through the business of living:

In the widest sense, health education may be defined as the sum total of all influences that collectively determine knowledge, belief and behaviour related to the promotion, maintenance and restoration of health in individuals and communities. These influences comprise formal and informal education in the family, in the school and in society at large, as well as in the special context of health service activities.

Although many would dispute this use of the term 'education' to cover such a wide range of learning experience (incidental as well as intentional), this exposition is valuable in a number of ways. It points to the wide range of arenas and circumstances in which influences on health may be exerted. It touches on the collective dimension of health (a community is, of course, more than just the sum of its individuals, and one person's actions may affect another's health; see Chapters 10 and 11). Furthermore, it embraces influences which are exerted without any health-related intent (which may be health-enhancing or health-damaging). Lastly, it brings to mind important, deliberately imposed influences which are not aimed at health enhancement: some are dressed up as being pro-health, but are in truth aimed at the promotion of something else (some materials produced by the dairy industry are an example); others concern the purposeful promotion of products, etc., which are patently damaging to health (tobacco advertising, for instance). Mike Daube (formerly Senior Lecturer in Health Education, University of Edinburgh) has referred to such efforts as '*pseudo-health education*' and '*anti-health education*', respectively.

Smith's broad interpretation thus serves as an important reminder of the background which must be recognized and addressed by the wide range of people who are concerned with the promotion of health through education. Clearly, however, it is purposefully provided pro-health education that is the main concern of this book, and henceforth the term 'health education' will be used in this context. We define this important subset of Smith's definition as follows:

Health education is communication activity aimed at enhancing positive health and preventing or diminishing ill-health in individuals and groups, through influencing the beliefs, attitudes, and behaviour of those with power and of the community at large.

Note the reference to power-holders in society. These include politicians, industrialists, and other people in business, and professionals within and outside the health service. This recognition that responsibilities in relation to health do not simply rest with 'the public' is a crucial and recurring theme of this book.

This must not be taken to suggest that the public at large is inevitably powerless. Helping people to greater control over their lives and health—empowerment—is a cardinal principle of health education, and indeed of health promotion as a whole (see p. 60).

Nor should the definition be construed as representing a 'top-down' or 'medically dominated' model. Two-way communication is envisaged, whereby those traditionally seen as 'providers' and 'recipients' learn from each other, and, as we shall now see, the '*beliefs, attitudes, and behaviour*' referred to above are broader in scope than might at first sight be assumed.

It should be noted that in the ensuing account 'beliefs' are dealt with separately from 'attitudes', for the sake of simplicity. The complex interrelationships between the two are discussed in Chapter 7.

3.1.1 Beliefs

A basic element in the shaping of beliefs is the acquisition of information, and the provision of 'health knowledge' is certainly a fundamental aspect of health education. The breadth of information relevant to health education is well seen in the 'tripartite typology' put forward by Draper *et al.* (1980) as follows.

— *Type 1 health education*: education about the body and how to look after it.
— *Type 2 health education*: provision of information about access to, and the most appropriate use of, health services.
— *Type 3 health education*: education about national, regional, and local policies and structures and processes in the wider environment which are detrimental to health.

As Draper and colleagues have pointed out, the first type is the commonest, and is indispensable for each new generation. Attention to the second has increased in recent times, but has rarely been manifested as an interactive process through which service providers may be educated by service users. The third type tends to be neglected, partly due to the fact that it leads to the path of greatest resistance (by powerful vested interests—see also p. 54), and partly as a result of the 'head-in-the-sand' attitude which denies that health has anything to do with politics.

The strength of a belief may be influenced by such factors as the credibility of an imparter of a 'message' (Section 7.4.1), the quality and appropriateness of communication (Section 7.4.2), the perceived relevance of a piece of information, and the extent to which a given belief fits in, or clashes, with existing beliefs (see also Section 7.4).

An illustration of human ability to insulate against uncomfortable or inconvenient beliefs is obtained from survey evidence that the majority of cigarette smokers believe that smoking is injurious to health, but that many also express the belief that their continuing to smoke would make no quantitative or qualitative difference to their future experience of illness, (OPCS 1983).

So far we have concentrated on beliefs directly concerning health or factors influencing it. The belief system germane to health education includes also beliefs about oneself: self concept is important in shaping perceptions as to one's ability to attain better health. For example, many people become conditioned to see themselves as being 'no good at sports' in such a way as to present a confidence barrier to taking adequate exercise.

3.1.2 Attitudes

Attitudes to health and to health-related factors, such as aspects of lifestyle, are considered in Chapter 7. Health educationists have in recent years been emphasizing the importance of the valuation of self concept—self-esteem—as a determinant of health. It has been concluded that people with a high level of self-esteem tend to be aware of their capabilities as individuals, to be relatively socially competent, and to have high resistance to (often unhealthful) pressures to 'conform'. On the other hand, low self-esteem has been linked to difficulties in establishing satisfactory relationships, vulnerability to pressures to conform, and feelings of a lack of control over life.

The situation is actually more complex than these generalizations imply. For example, research among schoolchildren has linked smoking in girls to negative body image (body image being a contributor to self-esteem), but has found smoking among 15–16 year-old males to be commoner in those with high self-esteem (Currie and Todd 1992). These findings represent associations between smoking status and self-esteem or body image: the directionality of the relationships cannot be inferred. Possible explanations for the apparent male paradox are that a high level of self-esteem enables individuals to resist what may now be a predominantly anti-smoking peer pressure, or that smoking is an effective prop for boys' self-esteem. Whatever the explanation, it can reasonably be argued that the fostering of self-esteem (through means which are not health-damaging) remains a legitimate objective for health education, especially since self-esteem contributes to true well-being (see p. 19). The practical implications of this argument are that everyone engaged in educating for health, whether doctors, nurses, school teachers, or others, should do everything possible to promote self-esteem, and must take great care that in-built aspects of their interactions with patients, students, clients, etc. (such as the inherent balance of power) are not allowed to erode it.

3.1.3 Behaviour

This element of the definition of health education naturally includes personal behaviour such as eating, drinking, smoking, and sexual conduct. In saying this, however, it is essential to point out that self-responsibility must be nurtured by helping people to develop health-related lifeskills, such as the ability to make decisions and to be assertive, rather than expecting them simply to take responsibility for their health. Similarly, the behaviour of power-holders, such as politicians and vested business interests, must be fully taken into account. In other words, combining these two points, care should be taken to avoid 'victim-blaming'.

The foregoing discussion is built on in later sections of this chapter, and in Part 2 of the book.

3.2 Who are the educators?

It will already have become apparent that many different categories of people can contribute to health education. The purpose of this section is to clarify the roles of the respective 'players' at national and local levels, including health education/promotion specialists.

The latter specialism has reflected the general shift in emphasis from health education to health promotion (see Chapter 4). Most of its practitioners are now referred to as health promotion officers or specialists, although the change in name has not uniformly been accompanied by a commensurate change in roles and responsibilities.

Health education/promotion specialists are employed by the National Health Service (NHS) in all parts of the UK, whether by health authorities/boards or, following the 'purchaser/provider split' created by health service reforms, in NHS trusts. There are also posts in some local authorities and some other agencies.

Health education at national level in the counties of the UK is the responsibility of the Health Education Authority in England, the Health Education Board for Scotland, Health Promotion Wales, and the Health Promotion Agency for Northern Ireland. All of these agencies are part of the NHS. Although some have health promotion rather than education in their name, the central function of all four organizations is health education, health promotion in the round (see Chapter 4) at national level being the province of central government. The educational role, however, is set within the context of health promotion, and includes advocacy and the giving of advice to policy-makers.

The most conspicuous part of health education is the high-profile mass media campaigns mounted by the national health education/promotion agencies and, increasingly, by medical charities and local health promotion services. The very prominence (and expense) of such campaigns can create excessive expectations (and even excessive reliance) on them. It is important to be realistic about what they can be looked upon to achieve. This question is considered in some detail on p. 135, but it is helpful to give brief clarification here.

Mass media initiatives, involving the use of television, for example, can be very effective in placing and maintaining health issues on the public agenda and in providing straightforward information. They are most likely to change attitudes in circumstances in which the audience is motivated towards such change; messages that are repeated or otherwise reinforced may in time contribute to a shift in societal values (Tones 1977). Mass media campaigns can enhance motivation to change behaviour. They can stimulate relatively simple, one-off behaviours on a mass scale (such as accepting immunization, or contacting a helpline) and they can trigger more complex behavioural change (for example, smoking cessation) in suitably primed individuals. The probability of mass behavioural change can be enhanced by providing support services (such as a smoking cessation telephone counselling service) and personal materials (for instance, a self-help guide to quitting smoking) (Donnan *et al.* 1994).

Whatever the nature of a mass media campaign, local health education efforts are vital (Tones 1983). This is well recognized by the UK national health education/promotion agencies, which direct much of their effort to supporting and facilitating grass-roots work. The educators at local levels are, potentially, everyone: every professional and lay person, and every agency in the community has a part to play in health education (and, more broadly, in health promotion—see Chapter 4), whether through formal or informal (including family and peer) networks and channels. The effectiveness of the overall health education effort in a given locality is, to a considerable degree, dependent on the extent to which potentials are realized. A crucial role of health promotion specialists working at local levels is to help others to develop the knowledge, attitudes, and skills they require to identify opportunities for health education/promotion, and to meet the challenges thus made apparent.

The remainder of this chapter presents a theoretical basis for health education, which can be applied by the full range of potential health educators in the community.

3.3 Approaches and ingredients

A large number of classifications and models of health education have been put forward in recent years. The details of these are of most relevance to specialists in the field. In this section and the next, two frameworks for analysis and action are outlined. It is intended that these be taken together with each other and with Chapter 4 in building up a feel for health education and its relationship to health promotion.

The first of these frameworks was developed jointly by a public health physician and a health education specialist with experience in working together (Tannahill and Robertson 1986).

Its origins lay in these authors' dissatisfaction with the way in which approaches to health education are commonly distinguished. Discussion often centres on rigidly demarcated 'models' of health education, such as 'medical', 'educational', and 'social' or 'political' models.

Such models tend to be looked upon in either or both of two ways:

(1) as indicative of both a professional and a philosophical understanding of health education, it being expected that a doctor or nurse would adhere to the medical model, a teacher to the educational model, and so on;

(2) as part of a developmental process, usually represented as a sequence from the medical to the educational model (reflecting the shift in the professional backgrounds of health education specialists from nursing to teaching), and often beyond to social or political perspectives (linked to further changes in the sources of health education/promotion specialists towards social sciences, etc.).

Both of these viewpoints are oversimplified and misleading. Indeed, they are potentially detrimental to the multidisciplinary practice of health education, through perpetuating counter-productive stereotypes and detracting from professional development and collaboration.

Health education theory and practice have always had medical, educational, and other components, and it is better to look at the evolutionary sequence in terms of changes in all of the various ingredients of the health education 'cake' and in the overall 'mix' than to sustain false distinctions between inevitably interlinking classical models.

Accordingly, approaches to health education may be classified as *traditional, transitional*, and *modern*.

3.3.1 Traditional approach (Fig. 3.1)

The traditional approach to health education has a negative focus, that is to say it is aimed fairly and squarely at prevention rather than addressing positive health.

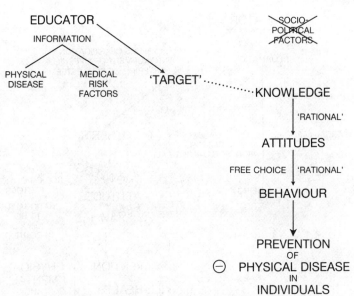

Fig. 3.1 Traditional approach to health education.

The main emphasis is on *physical* aspects of ill-health. This is reflected in the information base used, which represents a highly limited medical perspective.

Similarly, the educational basis is narrow. *Information* is provided by *educators* in the expectation of an *orderly sequence* from knowledge through attitudes to (medically defined) 'correct' behaviour. The notion of 'rational man' is implied.

Social and political determinants of health are neglected. People are considered to be *free to choose* their health-related behaviour.

Efforts are directed at *targeted individuals*. The collective dimension of health is not addressed.

3.3.2 Transitional approach

Recognition that the idea of a straightforward knowledge—attitudes—behaviour sequence was misguided led to a move towards manipulative, 'irrational' tactics, using lurid images with the intention of shocking or scaring people into behaving 'sensibly'. Such unlikely images as skulls smoking cigarettes were presented to the public, to very limited effect. Skull and crossbones imagery has even come to be used in the packaging and promotion of a brand of cigarettes.

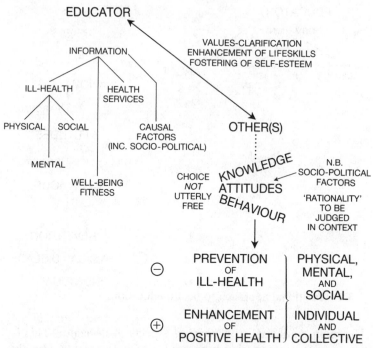

Fig. 3.2 Modern approach to health education.

3.3.3 Modern approach (Fig. 3.2)

This approach is more cumbersome to represent diagrammatically as it takes into account the complexity of health and the factors which influence it, and of modern educational theory and practice.

It can seen from Fig. 3.2 that the modern approach to health education is explicitly aimed not only at prevention but also at the promotion of *positive health*.

Furthermore, both positive and negative dimensions of health are seen as having *physical, mental* and *social* facets (in accordance with Chapter 2). This leads to a widening out of the 'content' of health education in line with the Draper *et al.* (1980) typology (see Section 3.1.1).

The educational framework is likewise broader, in acceptance of the abundant evidence that mere provision of information is not enough, that there is no tidy and inevitable step-wise progression from knowledge through attitudes to behaviour. The educational process here includes helping people to clarify their values (in relation to themselves, health, health-influencing behaviour, etc.; see also Chapter 9) and to acquire various *lifeskills* (see p. 31), with an emphasis on fostering their *self-esteem*.

Linked to this, the education process is *participatory*. Communication is *two-way*. The 'educator' ensures that the other(s) are able to express their knowledge and opinions, and respects and values these. In this way an understanding of people's perspectives, based on their life experiences, may be obtained, this being infinitely preferable to assaulting people with unsympathetic views of 'correctness' dependent on a medical judgement of 'rationality' (see also Chapter 7).

The principles of participation and two-way communication are easily seen as being applicable to face-to-face health education on a one-to-one or group basis. They should also, however, be followed when embarking on initiatives which involve high-profile mass media work or publications, in that there should be rigorous pre-testing of concepts and materials with the 'target groups' so that their perspectives may be brought to bear on the developmental process.

Major *constraints to freedom of choice* in health-related behaviour are acknowledged. The effects of socio-political factors on health are recognized, and efforts are made to secure a climate more conductive to good health (see also pp. 43, 59, and 60).

Collective dimensions to health, behaviour, and health education are seen as important.

A developmental sequence has been presented, but it has to be admitted that practice has not uniformly kept pace with principles. In schools, for instance, a great deal of sound curriculum development work has yet to reach many classrooms. Nevertheless, there has been encouraging progress in the UK over the last decade across the spectrum of arenas in which health education takes place.

A continued increase in awareness of the modern approach amongst the many occupational groups with a part to play will accelerate progress in health education, both through the direct benefits of various disciplines' pulling together and through further encouragement of an environment which facilitates the activities and proper development of specialist health education/promotion services.

Key aspects of the approach advocated will become clearer

on reading the next section, following which the implications for practice will be explored. Before moving on to the next theoretical framework, however, it is helpful to look in more detail at the question of freedom of choice, using cigarette smoking as an illustration.

Doctors, nurses, and others still often speak and act as though smokers are stupid people who have freely opted for a course of action which stands a high chance of making them ill and shortening their lives. Indeed this attitude has come to be taken as far as questioning smokers' rights for free treatment under the National Health Service. Committed smokers themselves, perhaps out of denial that they can be controlled by 'the dreaded weed', frequently collaborate in the perpetuation of such victim-blaming by insisting that they have freely and willingly chosen to smoke.

Imagine a society in which there is no mythological imagery surrounding cigarette smoking: no spurious association with manliness, elegance, sophistication, achievement, 'grown-upness', smartness, and so on; where there is open portrayal in tobacco advertising (if it exists at all) that cigarettes are dirty and smelly, and that smoking kills around one in seven of the total population; where there are sound, substantial, and co-ordinated health education programmes from cradle to grave; where it is acknowledged that tobacco does not soothe the nerves until one is already 'hooked' on it; where no other false values are attached to smoking; and where there are no social pressures to smoke. Suppose that in this environment an adult wakes up one day and announces that, having weighed up all the pros and cons, he or she has arrived at the unfettered decision to take up smoking 20 cigarettes daily for life, thereby running a one in four risk of dying prematurely. One might reasonably say that that person has freely chosen to smoke (or else question his or her sanity).

Real life is, of course, very different. False images and distorted values in relation to smoking are nurtured by misleading, sophisticated advertising campaigns, through sponsorship of sport and the arts, by other means of media portrayal (for instance in 'soap operas'), by peer pressure ('if you don't smoke you're a wimp', etc.), by role models, and so on. Moreover, decisions to start smoking are generally taken by minors (whom society considers to have little competence to make other important decisions). Also, of course, the practice is habit-forming. As McKeown (1976) pointed out so elegantly: 'Our habits commonly begin as pleasures of which we have no need and end as necessities in which we have no pleasure.' Add to all this the relationship between smoking and socio-economic disadvantage, and we have powerful arguments that the concept of freedom of choice in this context is seriously flawed, somewhat offensive, and rather dangerous. Some or all of these arguments apply to many other aspects of health-related behaviour, as diverse as taking other drugs (such as alcohol and illicit substances), eating, and even driving (witness the growth of a 'speed' culture, fuelled by the aggressive marketing of high-performance cars, and advertisements such as the one which invited us to 'test fly one tomorrow').

3.4 Orientations

The framework presented in the previous section serves to broaden views on how an individual or a particular profession, might go about educating for health (and being educated for health). Another way of examining the evolution of health education will now be outlined. It has implications for the way in which health education programmes should be planned and organized (see p. 6), but also serves to reinforce in a practical way theory presented in the foregoing account. This framework involves categorization of health education according to how efforts are orientated.

3.4.1 Disease-orientated (Fig. 3.3)

Despite improvements in the 1990s, this type of health education is still commonly endorsed, explicitly or implicitly, by politicians, epidemiologists, and health service managers.

Efforts are aimed at the prevention of specific diseases, and there is much emphasis on gauging success in terms of progress towards target rates of morbidity and mortality. The inherent assumption is that major preventable diseases, such as cardiovascular disorders and malignancies, are best dealt with by specific preventive programmes aimed at reducing relevant 'risk factors' (factors which confer an increased likelihood of developing particular diseases).

Fig. 3.3 Disease-orientated health education (CHD = coronary heart disease).

The focus is thus negative. People are expected to 'look after themselves' in the light of anti-cancer 'campaigns' and the like. This kind of approach is of limited educational validity. It is true that people who are already primed to make changes, such as stopping smoking or cutting down on alcohol, may well do so as a result of negatively focused anti-tobacco or anti-alcohol publicity or advice, but it is arguably unrealistic to expect wholesale changes in lifestyle as a result of purely preventively focused education. After all, why should we expect people to give up valued practices (for example, smoking, drinking to excess, eating too many chips, or simply being slothful), or embark on new ones which are perceived as nasty or even painful (such as eating a healthful diet or taking exercise), on the strength of some speculative, intangible future benefit?

This question becomes particularly pressing when one considers those in society who have the greatest health needs, for whom the present is a bitter struggle, pleasures are few (and often damaging), and there is little perception of a future worth investing in, or indeed even open to personal influence. It is also very relevant in relation to young people, who are insulated by time from a sharp focus on their own mortality (Tannahill 1992).

Further problems arise from the incrementalist nature of this approach to formulating health education programmes. What tends to happen is that individuals or groups work on single topics in relative, or even absolute, isolation from one another. Turning to the examples in Fig. 3.3, then, we may find that there is in a single community a coronary heart disease (CHD) prevention programme, one aimed at preventing cancers, and another concerned with dental disease. Given the overlap in risk factors for many types of disease (see Fig. 3.3), there will inevitably be considerable duplication of effort, which, as well as being wasteful, may lead to over-saturation and a community 'switch-off' response. Worse still, there is a considerable propensity for inconsistency of 'messages'. For instance, 'CHD preventers' may throw up their hands in horror at dental colleagues who may encourage children to eat fatty, salty crisps (rather than sugary snacks). Such professional inconsistency leads to public—and indeed professional—confusion and militates against beneficial changes in public behaviour and professional practice.

Another source of potentially damaging inconsistency lies in the scope there is for pragmatism to be eclipsed by epidemiological purity: trivial scientific nit-picking and professional point-scoring may distract from large areas of consensus (CHD prevention being a case in point).

Criticism can also be levelled at the fact that this is an 'expert-dominated' orientation. To draw an analogy with clinical practice, health professionals provide population 'diagnoses' and mass 'prescriptions'—without any community 'consultations'. Ordinary people are expected to 'comply' even though they may not agree with the diagnoses or see the prescriptions as being appropriate.

Most fundamentally, the disease-oriented model is unacceptably deficient in its incomplete view of health, not only in neglecting social and collective aspects but also in ignoring the positive dimension.

3.4.2 Risk factor-orientated (Fig. 3.4)

This is aimed at eliminating particular risk factors in order to prevent associated diseases. Much health education is currently focused in this way.

The main advantage of this approach over the disease orientation is in the recognition that a single risk factor can be linked to more than one disease category. With reference to examples shown in Fig. 3.4, a smoking prevention programme can stress associations with lung and other cancers, as well as CHD (and, of course, chronic bronchitis, emphysema, etc.); efforts can be directed at encouraging a low-risk diet, taking into account the many and

varied links between food and ill-health. Thus, although the
model is still an incrementalist one, there are fewer problems
with duplication and confusion.

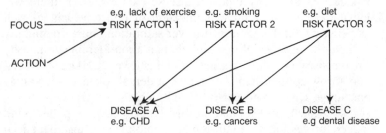

Fig. 3.4 Risk factor-orientated health education (CHD = coronary
heart disease).

However, the model is open to the other criticisms levelled at
disease-orientated health education: the view of health is inadequate; educational soundness is limited; and experts dominate.
Indeed the two orientations taken together are clearly reminiscent
of the 'traditional approach' to health education described earlier
(see p. 34).

3.4.3 Health-orientated (Fig. 3.5)

Here there is a dual focus: the aim is to enhance positive health as
well as to prevent ill-health. The physical, mental, and social components of both of these dimensions of health are recognized.

This is not to deny the importance and motivating qualities of
preventive benefits. It is simply an acknowledgement that the
incorporation of a positive focus enhances educational validity.
People are more likely to adopt a particular lifestyle if it appears
attractive. For instance, a healthful diet is presented as rich, varied,
and enjoyable, rather than as something Calvinistic and inevitably
less palatable than 'chips with everything'. Similarly, exercise is
promoted largely on the grounds that it makes people feel good,
instead of being painted as a painful chore. Health gain in terms of
well-being and fitness takes its place alongside preventive benefits,
and the balance of attention to the positive and the negative
dimensions can be varied according to the socio-economic status
or age of the 'target' population group (see p. 40) or other relevant
circumstances.

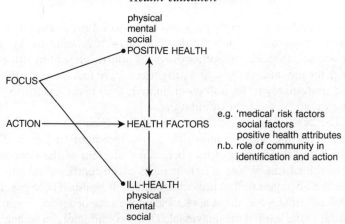

Fig. 3.5 Health-orientated health education.

Such an outlook is only common sense when we think of our own motivations in life. We like to do things which are appealing and enjoyable, and which give us tangible and relatively fast benefits; if at the same time we are increasing our chances of avoiding illness or premature death, then so much the better. A moment's thought as to how potentially damaging products and practices are promoted further reinforces the argument (think, for example, of advertisements linking alcohol with glamour, sophistication, and success, with no hint of the possibility of making a fool or nuisance of oneself socially, or of the impairment of performance which comes with inappropriate use; see also p. 38).

It should be noted that Fig. 3.5 refers to 'ill-health' rather than diseases. This acknowledges the need to go beyond the technical notion of disease (see Chapter 2). The distinction can be illustrated by referring to the fact that a relatively high proportion of medical consultations are, in doctors' eyes, trivial or even unnecessary, whereas presenting patients may feel otherwise. Another example is that someone may experience a level of mental ill-health which is highly significant to his or her life, even if it falls short of qualifying for a medical label as a psychiatric illness.

The 'health factors' referred to naturally do include 'medical' risk factors, but they go beyond these. Instead of dealing with individual aspects of lifestyle *in vacuo*, the model properly acknowledges underlying circumstances, including social factors. Common links in the origins of many types of health-damaging behaviour are recognized—for example peer and other social pressures (such as those arising out of multiple deprivation)—in relation to the use of alcohol, tobacco, and other drugs. A holistic view of health and its determinants prevails, and programmes are less incrementalist, and more likely to be well co-ordinated, than is the case with the disease and risk-factor orientations.

The health factors include also attributes discussed earlier in the account of the 'modern approach' to health education (see p. 37), and in the clarification of the 'behaviour' element of the definition of health education (see p. 31), qualities which contribute directly to true well-being as well as protecting against ill-health. These positive health attributes are just as applicable on the scale of a whole community as at the level of the individual. Thus a community can be helped to acquire a higher level of self-esteem and a set of empowering skills, skills which help it to take greater control both over its health as a collective entity and over that of its individual members.

Such considerations are consistent with recent interest within health promotion in the 'salutogenesis' approach (Antonovsky 1987), whereby efforts are directed towards identifying those factors which enable individuals and communities to attain and maintain good health in the face of many and wide-ranging hazards. There is a need for more research into the determinants of good health (Kelly 1989).

The principles set out here are central to the so-called community development approach to health. So also is another feature of the health-orientated model, namely community sensitivity and participation. Rather than operating purely on a professionally set agenda, the public, whether individually (for example in doctor–patient consultations) or collectively (for instance as part of a community of individuals) are involved in identifying health factors and priorities, and in shaping and securing action. Sensitivity and participation are likewise very important when working with individuals and small groups.

3.5 Communication

Although there are clear areas of overlap between the two theoretical frameworks put forward in this chapter, their practical implications differ to an extent, as has already been indicated. The health education 'approaches' framework has an important bearing on the way in which individual health educators and professional groups (doctors, nurses, environmental health officers, teachers, etc.) operate—and in particular communicate. The set of health education 'orientations', whilst impinging in a similar way on individual practice, is of greatest significance in relation to the planning of programmes of health education for a community (Tannahill 1990).

Programme planning is best considered in relation to the wider framework of health promotion, and is addressed in Chapter 4. The remainder of this chapter is concerned with communication.

The importance of two-way communication in health education was stressed in the account of the 'modern' approach to health education. Only through a participatory process may health professionals and other potential health educators find out what makes their 'clients' tick. Only thus may the educators avoid falling into the trap of imposing on the clients an inappropriate, professionally defined model of 'rationality'.

Consider the situation of a woman, pregnant for the seventh time. The family struggles to exist on State benefits, in the absence of paid employment. To the doctor confirming this latest pregnancy, the addition of yet another mouth to feed and body to clothe might well appear irrational. To the mother-to-be, the pregnancy may be highly valued: her six existing children might all be girls or boys, and she may yearn for a child of the other sex; alternatively, motherhood might be the only aspect of her life which has made her feel important and fulfilled. Who is the more 'rational'—the woman or her doctor?

The above illustration is, of course, something of a caricature of what in reality can be much more subtle contrasts between professional and lay perspectives. These differences can only be teased out through a 'partnership' (rather than 'provider–recipient') model of communication. In adopting this style of interaction, any 'messages' subsequently 'delivered' by the professional are more likely to be—and be perceived as—relevant to the 'client', and are thus more likely to be acted upon. The attendant treating of adults as adults, and of people's views as important rather than insignificant, helps to encourage 'adult' behaviour and fosters self-esteem.

To what extent does this model prevail in practice? An important study towards answering this was carried out in a general medical practice setting, but is undoubtedly relevant to a wide range of professionals. The 'Patient Project', carried out by the Health Education Studies Unit (1982) for the then Health Education Council, involved an intensive study of a large number of GP consultations. The aim was to explore how health education could facilitate public participation in informed debate about health issues. A number of the findings were favourable and highlighted the scope for informed decision-making and the sharing of lay and medical viewpoints. However, there was little to suggest that this potential was being tapped. Problems were found to arise from doctors' failing to explore patients' thinking frameworks, and a particularly notable finding was a tendency for the atmosphere in consultations to take a turn for the worse when patients sought to participate rather than be passive junior partners.

These findings are perhaps understandable, given the pedagogic way in which medical students and doctors are taught, and taught to teach. This does not, however, make the problems any less critical. One has to take very seriously the conclusions of the researchers that opportunistic health education by GPs might be dangerous as things stand, and that efforts should be concentrated on helping practitioners to develop core communication skills, rather than on specific aspects of health education and prevention.

It has to be acknowledged that medical schools and GP vocational training schemes have recognized the need for communication training. However, it is fair to say that there has, on the whole, been too little attention to the incorporation of lay feedback into such training.

Attempts to develop communication skills must give due recognition to the subtlety and complexity of the communication process. An understanding of some of the most significant pitfalls may be gained by breaking the process up into a number of stages.

Let us consider one side of a two-way interaction—communication from a doctor to a patient. This component of the communication process may be simplified as a sequence as follows.

Delivery → receipt → comprehension → interpretation

The extent to which information delivered is received is influenced by the quantity and concentration of information given, and by the language used. The doctor's language may be alien to the patient, not just because of professional jargon but also on account of social class and general educational differences. At a simpler level, of course, receipt is affected also by volume and clarity of enunciation, coupled with acuteness of hearing.

Comprehension following successful delivery and receipt of words is also critically affected by language. It is helpful for the doctor to check comprehension. However, even if this is done, and both doctor and patient are happy that a message has been given and successfully received, the interpretation of that message by the patient (and hence subsequent action) may well be seriously different from that intended by the doctor. Interpretation is influenced by linguistic factors and by thinking frameworks.

The distinction between comprehension and interpretation may be demonstrated through an exaggerated scenario, as follows. Suppose a doctor gives a woman a packet of oral contraceptives, telling her that if she takes them she will not become pregnant. The woman might 'understand' the instructions but interpret them as meaning that the packet is in some way a talisman controlling fertility, such that the act of taking the pills from the doctor (rather than ingesting them) is the crucial contraceptive step.

In checking understanding, then, asking the question 'Do you understand?' is not enough: interpretation must be properly ascertained, and patients' thinking frameworks (which may differ substantially from those of professionals) explored.

Superimposed on the above sequence, and having a bearing on the consequences of an episode of communication, is the question of retention of information. The quality of recall by patients has been found to be a barrier to subsequent action by some researchers (Ley *et al.* 1976), but did not seem to be a major problem in the Patient Project. Nevertheless, professionals must endeavour to ensure that their communication style makes for good retention.

In moving beyond the communication sequence, two further steps may be defined—intention and action. Behavioural intention following an interaction is determined, in part, by the elements considered above—language, understanding, retention, etc. Perceived relevance is also significant: 'messages' must be couched in an appropriate way, based on a knowledge of the patient's background and thinking framework. Justification by the professional of recommended action, in line with this thinking framework, is important in motivational terms.

Even then there may well be barriers to desired action, perhaps economic, social, or related to dependence. The professional must acquaint him/herself with these barriers, so that the patient can see that his/her position is well understood, and in order to work with the 'client' towards overcoming the obstacles.

So far we have concentrated on the verbal aspects of communication. It is, however, well known that non-verbal communication is vitally important. Returning once more to the GP situation, keeping a patient waiting, avoiding eye contact, prematurely writing a prescription, appearing distracted or uninterested, having a patronizing demeanour, or presenting a cluttered desk as a barricade may well detract utterly from even the most skilful use of words.

Doctors and other professionals have an advantage in the non-verbal area as regards the credibility and importance emanating from professional power. Another, more personal, type of power which may impinge on an interaction is charismatic power. Even the perceived attractiveness of a communicator may have significant effects. Finally, communication is more likely to be successful if the 'client' sees that the professional has some important characteristics in common with him/herself, although genuine empathy can make up for a lack of this (see also Section 7.4.1).

It is important to recognize that the above represents an analysis of one side of the process of communication. The factors and elements described and discussed operate also in the other direction, from 'client' to professional. The purpose of spelling this out is not to overwhelm the reader with the convolutions of communication (the problems *can* be overcome), but rather to stress once more the importance of a participatory, two-way model of communication.

Although the emphasis in this account has been on one-to-one communication, the same basic principles hold for individuals or teams of professionals working with groups or whole communities.

3.6 Conclusions

1. Health education seeks to enhance positive health and to prevent or diminish ill-health, through influencing beliefs, attitudes, and behaviour. The stimulation of a healthful environment—social and political as well as physical—is an important objective.
2. Health education must reach power-holders in society rather than just

the general public. Moreover, it must contribute to the empowerment of ordinary members of the community, through developing lifeskills and fostering self-esteem.

3. Mass media initiatives are of value, but community-based work is vital.

4. Everyone has a part to play in health education and, more broadly, in health promotion. Health promotion specialists can help others to identify and develop their roles.

5. Traditional, transitional, and modern approaches to health education may be distinguished. Practice has not uniformly kept pace with advances in theory.

6. The modern approach uses a broad information base and sound educational principles, and recognizes the importance of socio-political factors in health and health-related behaviour. It is a participatory model and has major implications for the way in which professionals should communicate with their 'clients'.

7. An evolutionary process in health education—from disease-orientated, through risk factor-orientated, to health-orientated—may be described. Once again we find that practice has lagged behind principles.

8. The health-orientated approach is preferable on both philosophical and organizational grounds. It has implications for programme planning.

4 Health promotion

Having explored the field of health education in some detail in Chapter 3, we shall now consider two more terms—'prevention' and 'health protection'—before moving on to define 'health promotion'.

4.1 Prevention

Central to prevention is the notion of reducing the risk of occurrence of a disease process, illness, injury, disability, handicap, or some other unwanted phenomenon or state. More detailed definition of the term is customarily left to its classification as 'primary', 'secondary', and 'tertiary', the value of which lies in its reminding us of the scope for prevention after the first onset of a particular health problem. Unfortunately there are a number of drawbacks associated with this nomenclature.

First, a review of the literature (Tannahill 1985a) indicates that there is no standard definition of the three levels of prevention: particulars differ significantly. A shorthand vocabulary in such a situation is thus unhelpful and hazardous: the labels 'primary', 'secondary', and 'tertiary' used alone, in the absence of unanimity of meaning, become worthless.

Secondly, the classification focuses on *disease*, the most glaring exclusion being the area of family planning, which most people would consider to be an important aspect of prevention (of social and mental ill-health, for instance).

Thirdly, the various schemes used include, whether by implication or explicit statement, *treatment* of ill-health. For example, 'secondary prevention' has been defined as 'the treatment and cure of established disease' (Alderson 1976). Thus just about everything a doctor does could be construed as prevention. It is self-evident that treatment is aimed at the prevention of certain consequences of ill-health (such as death), but the blurring of distinctions between prevention and cure and palliation in this way is undesirable: it renders meaningless present-day political and professional rhetoric in favour of prevention.

The benefits of the traditional approach to classification can be preserved, and the problems lessened, by discarding convenient tags which allow us to speak without making our meanings clear (even to ourselves), and describing instead four foci for prevention, as follows.

1. *Prevention of the onset or first manifestation of a disease process, or some other first occurrence, through risk reduction.* Taking coronary heart disease as an illustration, this includes efforts to avoid high blood cholesterol levels, to discourage smoking, and to maintain or secure an adequately low blood pressure. Accident prevention through reducing hazards or risk-taking behaviour is another example. Broadened out from matters of disease, this category includes, for example, the avoidance of a first unwanted pregnancy through contraception.

2. *Prevention of the progression of a disease process or other unwanted state, through early detection when this favourably affects outcome.* In relation to disease, this includes methods of picking up precursor or presymptomatic stages of particular conditions (such as screening for premalignant changes in the cervix and for early breast cancer, respectively). Although the treatment of discovered abnormalities is clearly an essential component, it is early detection that is the true preventive step. Returning to the case of pregnancy, detection of unintended conception or an abnormal fetus at a stage early enough to consider termination fits here.

3. *Prevention of avoidable complications of an irreversible, manifest disease or some other unwanted state.* In the interests of meaningful and commonsense distinction between prevention and treatment, this excludes, for example, the medical or surgical management of angina or the control of blood glucose levels in diabetes. Measures aimed at minimizing indirect consequences of an illness are, on the other hand, included—an example being attempts to prevent pressure sores or urinary tract infections in multiple sclerosis. Arrangements for the adoption of an unwanted child might be included here.

4. *Prevention of the recurrence of an illness or other unwanted phenomenon.* Examples include efforts to prevent a second heart attack or unwanted pregnancy.

It has to be admitted that this system of classification is less than ideal. Perfection is impossible to achieve when seeking to reduce the continua of diseases' natural histories to a set of man-made compartments, and distinctions between prevention and treatment, however desirable, are inevitably arbitrary and superficial. Nevertheless, it is hoped that the essence of the philosophy and practice of prevention can be gleaned from it and that at least the reader has been made aware of the undesirability of loose use of vocabulary against such a complex background.

Given the existence of a number of excellent publications dealing with the subject, it is not intended to go into the principles of preventive medicine any further in this book, except to examine criteria for screening (see p. 143).

4.2 Health protection

This can be seen as the descendant of the great old regulatory public health measures which have had such an impact on the population's health over the last century. It may be defined as follows.

Health protection comprises legal or fiscal controls, other regulations and policies, and voluntary codes of practice, aimed at the enhancement of positive health and the prevention of ill-health.

Health protection makes it less likely that people will encounter hazards in the environment, and that they will behave in an unhealthful manner, while increasing their chances of living in a positively healthful environment and having a lifestyle which promotes positive health. (It is the wider environment—political, legislative, social, etc., as well as physical—which is referred to here.) In other words, it is about making healthy choices easier choices.

The concept, and barriers to regulatory action, will now be illustrated through a series of examples, following which ethical considerations will be briefly explored.

4.2.1 Legal control

Examples include legislation concerning: the wearing of seat-belts in cars; the sale of alcohol and tobacco to minors; drinking and driving; the control of communicable diseases; and health and safety at work.

4.2.2 Fiscal control

An example of pro-health fiscal policy in the UK is the imposition of differential taxation on petrol to make the unleaded variety cheaper, as an inducement to conversion to this type of fuel in the interest of environmental protection.

An inverse link between the consumption of tobacco and its price in real terms is well-recognized (ASH *et al.* 1988), and the UK Government has given a commitment to increasing tobacco duties by, on average, at least 3 per cent in real terms each year (Department of Health 1994).

Although, unlike tobacco, alcohol is not, in epidemiological terms, harmful at all levels of usage (and indeed moderate drinking may, overall, confer health benefits), it is widely accepted that the extent of alcohol-related problems in a society correlates with per capita consumption. An inverse price/consumption relationship has been demonstrated for alcoholic drinks (FCM 1988), even among problem drinkers (Kendell *et al.* 1983). However, there is as yet in the UK no commitment to increases in alcohol duty, and the real price of alcoholic drinks falls from time to time. More generally, there is no coherent policy of differential taxation of goods and services according to whether they promote or damage health.

4.2.3 Other regulations and policies

Regulatory action is not the exclusive province of central government. In recent years, for example, many employers (including health authorities/boards, who have a special exemplar role) have developed policies to promote non-smoking on their premises. Workplace policies on alcohol and problem drinking have also been becoming more common, as have food and health policies.

So far we have concentrated on specific hazards, such as tobacco and alcohol. We should, however, remember that more fundamental aspects of public policy-making, such as those relating to housing, transport, education, employment, and the prevention and alleviation of poverty, impinge on health. Health protection policies can, and must, address the full range of 'prerequisites for health' as identified by WHO (p. 68).

4.2.4 Voluntary codes

These are in general poor substitutes for compulsion. The promotion and advertising of cigarettes in the UK, for instance, is regulated by a process of agreement between the tobacco industry and the Government, and breaches of the resulting voluntary code have been so frequent, and in many instances so crass, as to become legendary (Roberts 1986, 1987). On the other hand, as has been reported by Government economic advisers, bans on tobacco advertising and promotion in other parts of the world have been linked to reductions in smoking (Department of Health 1992*a*).

4.2.5 Barriers to health protection

A major barrier to national regulatory action in favour of health appears to be a simple process of neglect—failure to look for, and give priority to, likely health consequences of public policy across a broad front. The 'Skoal Bandits' affair (p. 101) is perhaps a demonstration of what can happen when there is no proper mechanism for gearing action by the various Departments of the Government towards the protection of the nation's health.

Another problem is perceived clashes of interest between Government Departments. Thus, it has been argued, deterrent increases in tobacco taxation are not overall in the national interest since tobacco revenue is the country's third largest source of income (after Value Added Tax and oil). In short, we cannot afford successfully to discourage smoking with any rapidity, especially as many more people might then live to collect their pensions.

This line of argument may be countered in three ways. First, an economic analysis of a package of anti-smoking measures (including a rise in duty), based on a predicted 40 per cent resultant reduction in smoking, has suggested that, as well as saving many lives and much misery, the measures would result in an increase in Government revenue income from the higher prices paid by the remaining smokers (Atkinson and Townsend 1977). Secondly, and more fundamentally, taxation is transferable: the same amount of revenue may be obtained by taxing something else (such as income), and so the case for the economic imperative of smoking is spurious. Thirdly, it is surely unacceptable for public policy (even if the economic reasoning were sounder) to preserve the status quo whereby one in seven deaths in England and Wales, for example, results from smoking. A national policy of compulsory euthanasia at retirement age would be a more honest, equitable, and effective means of achieving the desired economic objective!

The third barrier to health protection nationally stems from the enormous power of vested interests over public policy-making. Big business is in a strong position to oppose pro-health policies and perpetuate unhealthful ones, in the interests of profit. It is widely stated that progress towards a sensible, coherent food policy, for instance, is persistently hampered by the influence of the food and agricultural industries.

The impact of Industry on policies which affect health is very clearly seen in relation to tobacco. The Zoos Bill episode of 1981 (Anonymous 1981) is a case in point. More than 100 amendments to this hitherto uncontroversial Private Member's Bill suddenly materialized, with the result that another Bill, aimed at giving the Government power to control tobacco promotion, ran out of Parliamentary time. The latter had been expected to gain a majority. The amendments to the Zoos Bill were tabled by a handful of Members of Parliament (MPs), one of the principal participants being a parliamentary adviser to a major tobacco company, and others also having direct or indirect links with the industry. Not surprisingly this incident has been seen as a case of filibustering (an obstruction of legislation through delaying tactics) in which health lost out to darker motives. This raises the question of links between MPs and vested interests which damage health. These may be directly financial (through appointments with tobacco, alcohol, or related public relations companies) or may involve constituency or trade union interests in industries. Contributions to political party funds might also be seen as potentially significant.

Political influence at the national level is reinforced by the power of vested interests over the public and the media. Power over the public is exerted by control over the availability and pricing of products for consumers (health education cannot succeed if advocated healthful goods cannot be found or afforded), by marketing strategies, and so on. Power over the media may take the form of lucrative advertising accounts 'with strings attached' (such as hints to magazines that business will be taken elsewhere if, say, anti-smoking features appear), of misinformation, and so forth.

These illustrations of constraints to health protection nationally are matched by interferences at more local levels. The raising of awareness of such local and national obstacles is an important component of type 3 health education as described by Draper *et al.* (1980) (p. 29). Given the enormity and power of the opposition it is easy to see why this type of work tends to be played down.

It is, however, heartening to see professional bodies, such as the

British Medical Association and the Royal College of Physicians of London, campaigning for health protection measures (BMA 1986).

4.2.6 Ethical considerations

In many instances, attempts are made to justify antipathy to health protection on ethical grounds. Thus, it is often argued, it would be wrong to exert compulsory control on tobacco advertising or sponsorship because people's freedom of choice would be restricted. The issue of free rational choice in health-related behaviour has already been considered in some detail (see p. 38), and on the basis of that discussion it is suggested here that the concept should be treated with scepticism. Failure to regulate powerful concerns which damage health serves to perpetuate the freedom of choice of those with a great deal of power (major business and others with vested interests in unhealthful products or activities) to exploit those with relatively little (the public).

In any case, society accepts a great deal of regulation for the common good: it is illogical that the manufacturers of cigarettes, the major preventable cause of serious illness and premature death, and alcohol, with its immense direct and indirect impact on social, mental, and physical health, should be treated so lightly (see Chapter 10). The contrast with the treatment of illicit drugs is striking; no-one, of course, makes a public case for the protection of heroin barons, for instance.

One specific ethical dilemma worth looking at here is the question of taxation of tobacco products. There is a widespread feeling among pro-health lobbyists in the UK that the Government's fiscal policy in this area does not go far enough, and indeed a number of agencies and individuals have called for much larger increments. A counter-argument to swingeing increases is that they would hit the poorest people most (see Marsh and McKay 1994). It would be desirable to have a public debate on the question of the degree to which fiscal action should be taken on tobacco. In the meantime it would seem reasonable to ensure that tobacco products do not become cheaper in real terms.

4.3 A model of health promotion

We are now, at last, in a position to reflect on the meaning of 'health promotion'. Although the term has been in existence for many years, it came to the fore during the 1980s, and since then has become increasingly fashionable in professional and political circles.

Given this popularity, it is most unfortunate that 'health promotion' is used in a number of different ways, even by the same people. The problem is accentuated by the fact that the term tends to be bandied about somewhat glibly, without clarification of underlying meanings. As with health education, therefore, it is perfectly possible—and indeed by no means uncommon—for two people, or even an entire committee or conference, to have a discussion about health promotion and be referring to very different things. In effect, health promotion has became a dazzling bandwagon, gaining momentum, and with all and sundry clamouring to climb aboard, without giving sufficient thought to what it is and where it is going.

It is helpful at this stage to look at a number of interpretations which have been put forward in recent years, nothing how these vary in scope and detail.

Health promotion has frequently been taken to cover attempts to promote positive health. This interpretation has often been implied rather than explicit: there has, for instance, been a tendency to talk or write of 'health promotion and disease prevention' as a sort of inseparable coupling, without making clear the perceived differences between the two expressions.

Some have made an explicit distinction between health promotion and prevention (NALGO 1984; WHO 1984; Nutbeam 1986). The value of this, however well-argued the case, is markedly diminished by the fact that most people would see health education as central to health promotion, and at the same time health education is still often treated largely (or even exclusively) as a subset of prevention. Moreover, research into what has been written and done by health promotion groups, professional bodies, etc. under that banner of health promotion reveals that preventive activities, such as immunization and screening, are highly prominent.

In practice, many people give the impression that they equate health promotion with health education. Even in the current vogue for health promotion, policy-makers and managers often seem to place an exclusive, or near-exclusive, emphasis on what are, in truth, educational interventions. The confusion has been aggravated by the near-wholesale change in name for specialist agencies and practitioners from health education to health promotion (p.

32). There is a need to preserve a distinction between the two terms, so that the non-educational elements of health promotion (p. 59) are properly pursued, while sound educational principles are brought to bear within the broader context.

Even more unsatisfactory is the interpretation of health promotion as a series of one-off 'glitzy' events. This arises from what we see as a misunderstanding of the 'promotion' component of the term as having to do with 'selling' health (as opposed to enhancing or nurturing it), and has at times gone as far as changing the term to 'health promotion*s*'. There is a place for high-profile and fun events, but we must not see them as the beginning and end of health promotion. More substance is required.

Other, fuller views of health promotion have been put forward. Thus the term has often been used as an 'umbrella' covering health education and 'social engineering' (through fiscal, legal, and other environmental manipulations) (Tones 1983). Where the term is used in this wider manner, health promotion is frequently defined as a list of ingredients, without examination of their interconnections.

It has even been commonplace to use such a broad interpretation as to imply that all activities which seek to improve health come under the heading of health promotion (Dennis *et al.* 1982). This is at best unhelpful and at worst damaging, in terms of fuzzing the necessary differentiation between powerful, established areas of health service provision and important alternative channels (still relatively neglected) for investment.

In recognition that 'health promotion' had acquired so many meanings as to become meaningless, and taking into account activities undertaken and papers written in the name of health promotion, Tannahill (1985*b*) developed a model of health promotion. It is intended as a framework for defining, planning, and 'doing' health promotion, and it has become widely adopted. The construct can now be described against the essential backdrop of our clarification of the meanings of related terms (Chapters 2 and 3, and pp. 50–6). According to the Tannahill model (Fig. 4.1), health promotion comprises three overlapping spheres of activity: *health education* (or, more precisely, that part which contributes to the overall goal of health promotion—see p. 52), *prevention* (p. 50), and *health protection* (p. 52).

Seven domains (numbered in the figure) may be distinguished within health promotion, as follows.

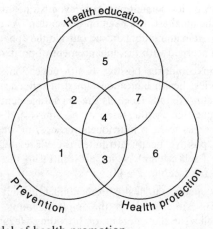

Fig. 4.1 A model of health promotion.

1. This domain includes preventive measures such as immunization and cervical screening (see pp. 51, 57). Hypertension case-finding, screening for handicapping congenital disorders, developmental surveillance, dental fissure sealing, and the use of nicotine-containing chewing gum to aid smoking cessation are other examples.

2. This includes educational efforts to influence lifestyle in the interests of preventing ill-health, as well as efforts to encourage the uptake of preventive services. In addition, the two-way nature of the educational process must not be forgotten: communication channels must be used to ensure that appropriate and desirable preventive services are provided (see pp. 29, 37, 44).

3. Numerous examples of preventive health protection have already been mentioned (pp. 52–4). Fluoridation of public water supplies to protect against dental disease is another. This overlap between prevention and health protection can be viewed in another way, as policy commitment to the provision of preventive measures such as those described under domain 1.

4. Preventive health protection measures cannot be relied upon simply to emerge spontaneously. Education of policy-makers is important. One of the most notable successes in this regard in the UK has been in the area of seat-belts: it having been demonstrated that public health education alone was ineffective as a means of securing widespread use of safety belts in motor vehicles, intense Parliamentary lobbying was rewarded by legislation. Efforts to stimulate a social environment which demands or accepts preventive health protection measures are also important. Once again, the overlap between spheres of the model may be looked at in a different way: thus this domain also

encompasses policy commitment to preventive health education.

[So far, the emphasis has been on prevention. As can be seen from Fig. 4.1, the remaining domains lie outside the sphere of prevention. They are concerned with the enhancement of positive health.]

5. This domain comprises positive health education, which falls into two categories: health education aimed at influencing behaviour on positive health grounds (such as the encouragement of a productive use of leisure time in the interests of fitness and well-being); and that which seeks to help individuals, groups, or whole communities to develop positive health attributes (health-related lifeskills and a high level of self-esteem), which are central to the enhancement of true well-being (see pp. 19, 43).

6. A positive dimension to health protection has already been mentioned (see p. 52). An example is the implementation of a workplace smoking policy in the interests of providing clean air. Another is the commitment of public funds to the provision of attractive and accessible leisure facilities in order to promote positive health.

7. This domain embraces raising awareness of, and securing support for, positive health protection measures, among the public and policy-makers. It also includes policy commitment to positive health education.

The domains have been presented in this way to demonstrate the wide range of possibilities for health promotion. They are not to be seen as occupying rigidly separate compartments: the model is not intended to be seen as a typology of health promotion. In particular, it has to be pointed out that the positive and preventive objectives, whether in health education or health protection, will in reality tend to be combined. The reasons for somewhat artificially separating the two in this account are that the positive dimension is in practice too easily lost and that in fact a good case can often be made for making the positive aim the primary one.

The following summary definition of health promotion arises out of the model presented here. (Note the incorporation, in modified form, of the goal of health promotion presented at the end of Chapter 2.)

Health promotion comprises efforts to enhance positive health and reduce the risk of ill-health, through the overlapping spheres of health education, prevention, and health protection.

The cardinal principle of health promotion thus defined is empowerment. Health education seeks to empower by providing necessary information and helping people to develop skills and a healthy level of self-esteem (see pp. 30, 37), so that they come to feel that significant control resides within themselves, rather than feeling buffeted about by external forces outside their sphere of influence. The provision of good preventive services and the shaping of a healthful environment through health protection also contribute to this process of empowerment.

4.4 Programme planning

Like health education, health promotion must be everybody's (and every body's—see Quigley 1981) business. At the same time, the health sector must be seen as having the lead role to play: it must be prepared to set a good example, to take a proactive part in securing alliances for health, and to play a catalytic and enabling role in the sense of helping others towards a commitment to, and capabilities in, health promotion.

In this section, the issue of planning for the 'delivery' of health promotion is dealt with from a health sector perspective. The issue under consideration is essentially that of how priorities for health promotion, such as those set out in central government policy documents (see Section 4.5.2) can be translated into effective and efficient programmes of action (a programme being defined as a coherent set of ongoing activities towards defined strategic objectives). A key challenge is to ensure that the approach adopted is one which will stimulate and support action across society as a whole, not just within health services.

4.4.1 Topic-based approach

Not unnaturally, national policy statements tend to identify as priorities major categories of health/ill-health (such as coronary heart disease, cancer, HIV/AIDS, dental/oral health, and accidents) and important health-related behaviours (for example, smoking, alcohol misuse, drug misuse, eating, and exercise). A common response by specialist health education/promotion organizations, whether operating at national or sub-national levels, has been to devise a programme for each health and behavioural topic—to have a coronary heart disease (CHD) programme, a cancer programme, a smoking programme, an alcohol programme, and so on (Fig. 4.2). This corresponds to a combination of disease- and risk factor-orientated health education as described in Chapter 3. There are serious problems with this approach (Tannahill 1994).

Fig. 4.2 Topic-based approach to programme planning.

The first, and most fundamental, problem emanates from the fact that there are extensive links between the topics. Overlaps in risk factors for many categories of ill-health were mentioned in Section 3.4.1. Moreover, a number of health-damaging behaviours have much in common with one another. A good illustration of both of these points is provided by alcohol misuse. It is a risk factor for a number of types of cancer and for hypertension (and thus CHD). It can lead to a number of dental/oral problems, including cancer and traumatic damage. Through loosening inhibitions, clouding judgement, and impairing the use of condoms, it predisposes to sexual conduct which carries a risk of HIV and other infections, and unplanned pregnancy. It is commonly implicated in accidents. As a behaviour, alcohol misuse shares a number of determinants with smoking and the use of illicit drugs; like these other behaviours, it can be habit-forming. Also, alcohol consumption has to be considered in relation to a healthy diet.

As indicated in Section 3.4.1, the overlaps between topics predispose to wasteful, and even counter-productive, duplication of effort. Co-ordination across topics is central to efficiency and effectiveness. With the best will in the world, adequate co-ordination is unlikely where programmes are topic-based: the individuals and teams responsible for such programmes tend to be very single-minded and even, in their enthusiasm for this area of concern, competitive with each other. It is illogical to deal with individual topics in absolute or relative isolation. Also, in any case, it is impossible to synthesize a full and coherent view of health and its determinants (see Section 3.4.3) from individual categories of health/ill-health and behaviour.

Another problem relates to the fact that topic-based programmes all need to reach the public through mass media and a range of settings and sectors—schools, health care settings, the workplace, other formal and informal community settings, and the voluntary sector. Put another way, they have to be active in a range of 'arenas', trying to help each arena to fulfil its health promotion potential (Fig. 4.3). This is a tall order for the programme managers or teams. Also, the principal qualities necessary to be an expert in a topic differ from those needed to deliver health promotion programmes. Topic specialists primarily need the investigative and analytical skills of the researcher, whereas programme delivery commands expertise in education, communication, networking, and project management.

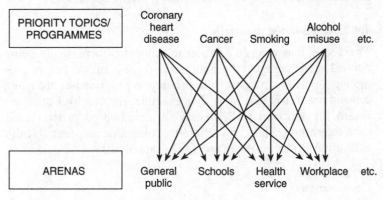

Fig. 4.3 Topic-based approach and arenas for health promotion.

So far, we have concentrated on problems from the point of view of the specialist health promotion organization. As pointed out by Tannahill (1994), it is necessary to consider also the perspectives of 'gate-keepers' to the various settings and sectors, whose active participation is essential for success. Such people include education authority representatives and officials, and head teachers of schools; hospital and primary care managers, doctors, and nurses; heads of industrial and commercial companies, workplace managers, and trade union officials; and workers in voluntary organizations. To them, topic-based programmes result in a feeling of being bombarded by a disjointed and incrementalist set of demands from various people. This is a classic example of 'top-downism', as opposed to the 'bottom-up' health promotion ethos (p. 68). Take school head teachers, for example. They will not consider it feasible to accommodate numerous new programmes into an already crowded curriculum. They are entitled to be disgruntled at having been excluded from early developmental stages. They are likely to be concerned that the topic-based approach is uncoordinated: their preference will almost certainly be for investment in an infrastructure and methodologies specifically geared to the school setting, health-orientated as opposed to disease- or risk factor-orientated (see Section 3.4), and ensuring appropriate educational inputs at the various stages of the school career. The undesirability of trying to incorporate a series of topic-based health promotion programmes into the curricula and extracurricular activities of schools is widely recognized, and comprehensive, co-ordinated schools programmes are established, or being established, in many countries.

4.4.2 Arena-based approach

The above reasoning in relation to schools is increasingly being applied more generally by national and sub-national health promotion agencies, so that health promotion programmes are being centred on arenas (Fig. 4.4). For example, the Health Education Board for Scotland (HEBS) has six arena-based programmes, each the responsibility of a different programme manager (Health Education Board for Scotland 1993; Tannahill 1994):

General public
Health service
Schools
Voluntary sector
Workplace
Community

Two arenas are worth clarifying at this point. The general public programme utilizes mass media to reach the general population or sub-groups thereof. It provides a highly visible backdrop for the work of other national, and sub-national, programmes. The community programme is concerned with community settings other than those covered by the other programmes. It involves working through existing formal and informal networks, and building new ones. It should be noted that the arena-based programmes are supplemented by a special projects programme, which enables HEBS to participate in national and international special projects (such as World AIDS Day, UK No Smoking Day), and gives flexibility to respond quickly to new challenges and opportunities.

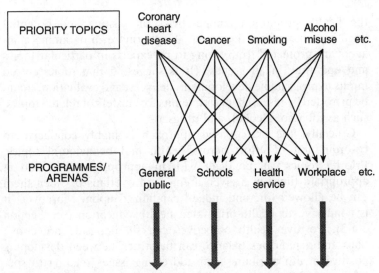

Fig. 4.4 Arena-based approach to programme planning.

The remit of HEBS is health education, and its programmes are health education programmes. However, the aim of each arena-based programme is to develop the full health promotion role of the arena in question. That is to say, the work involves educating for health promotion. For example, the schools programme is set within the concept of the health promoting school (SHEG and SCCC 1990; WHO, Council of Europe, and Commission of the European Communities 1993), encouraging attention to the general school ethos and environment, and to extracurricular activities, as well as to the curriculum (see also Section 6.5). A focus on arenas is appropriate also for organizations with a fuller health promotion remit.

The arena-based approach confers benefits which are essentially the mirror image of the disadvantages of the topic-based approach (Tannahill 1994). It facilitates national–local collaboration, and enables health promotion agencies together to permeate the community, reaching people wherever they are, and developing appropriate infrastructures in the arenas. The approach allows professionals and others in the various arenas to contribute their experience and expertise to programme development and implementation, thus promoting a feeling of 'ownership' among key players and enhancing responsiveness to community needs. It facilitates the provision of education and training to help develop the health promotion competencies of existing and potential 'health promoters' in the arenas. Furthermore, programme managers are protected from trying to be experts in particular topics and operating in all arenas. (It is suggested that topic-centred inputs to programme development, delivery, and evaluation should be provided by researchers with remits for clusters of related topics, such as tobacco, alcohol, and drugs.)

Crucially, the arena-based approach is highly conducive to co-ordination of effort across health and behavioural topics. Priority topics can be dealt with in appropriate ways and at appropriate times in a given arena, and overlaps between them can be allowed for, and indeed capitalized upon. Moreover, it is conducive to health-orientated health education (see Section 3.4.3). Positive health objectives can sit alongside preventive ones and a judicious balance can be struck between developing positive health attributes and addressing issues relating to specific topics. Through co-ordination across programmes, general public programme activities can be reinforced as appropriate in settings and sectors, while the 'bottom-up' dynamic in other programmes enables setting- and sector-specific needs to be identified and met.

Returning to health promotion more broadly, the arena-based approach allows for the dovetailing of co-ordinated and comprehensive health education work in particular community settings with specific preventive services and health protection measures, tailored to the needs and opportunities presented by the particular settings (see Sections 6.4 and 6.5 for examples). Setting-based preventive services and health protection policies have, of course, to be backed by planning and co-ordination on a national scale, just as local-level health education should complement national educational initiatives.

In addition to topics and arenas, two other dimensions have to be considered: groups and localities.

Arena-based programmes must actively address differences in health needs and required health promotion approaches between various population groups (such as young people, old people, women, men, and ethnic minorities). Just as it is necessary to co-ordinate work on particular topics across arenas, it is important to ensure a coherent approach to specific groups through an overview of programmes and collaboration between programme managers.

There is a widespread move towards planning health services on a locality basis. The arenas model of health promotion planning is applicable at the level of small community patches, not just countries, areas, or districts. Professionals and others, including community representatives, can work as teams seeking to make the most of the health promotion opportunities in a patch through the various arenas, supported by arena-centred programme development at district, area, and national levels. We look on locality planning and purchasing of services as having an exciting potential for the furthering of community-sensitive health promotion.

4.5 Wider contexts

4.5.1 Health promotion and Health for All

At the Thirtieth World Health Assembly in 1977, the attainment of health for all was accepted as the main social target of governments and the World Health Organization in the remaining years of the century. The strategy for 'Health for All by the Year 2000' (now as the end of the century approaches, referred to as 'Health for All') gained momentum with the Declaration of Alma Ata in 1978, and took further shape in Europe in 1985, with the publication of a book setting out the principles and identifying 38 targets (WHO 1985). The UK Government has expressed strong support for the strategy. The targets have since been updated (WHO 1991).

Although the vocabulary used by WHO (WHO 1984) in relation to health promotion and prevention is different from that used in delineating health promotion in this chapter (indeed it is unsatisfactory in a number of respects: Tannahill 1985b), it is clear from the Health for All strategy that all aspects of health promotion as defined here are considered to be vital in pursuing better health for everyone. As well as legitimizing health promotion, the strategy is centred on certain key principles which are of major relevance to work in this field.

First, as befits a strategy for health for *all*, the promotion of equity in health is a central principle. Health promotion must seek to redress inequalities in health by encouraging equity of opportunity to enjoy good health. Secondly, the impact on health of policies and services outside the health sector is stressed. This is well seen in the identified *prerequisites for health*, which have major implications for health protection (see pp. 52–3):

Freedom from the fear of war
Equal opportunity for all
Satisfaction of basic needs
— food
— basic education
— water and sanitation
— decent housing
— secure work and a useful role in society
Political will and public support

Related to this, Health for All emphasizes the need for fruitful intersectoral collaboration. The importance of multidisciplinary collaboration is similarly highlighted. These principles are crucial to health promotion, and there is increasing attention globally to the development of 'healthy alliances' ('alliances for health' being a more apposite term).

Finally, community participation in matters affecting their health (a 'bottom-up' approach) is an essential feature of the strategy, and of health promotion.

Primary care and health promotion may be seen as 'twin pillars' of the Health for All strategy (Tannahill 1988*a*). It makes good sense to try to strengthen the bridging between these pillars by further developing health promotion in the primary care setting (see Section 6.4).

Under the Health for All umbrella, WHO has published a number of statements on the principles of health promotion. Most notable among these is the 'Ottawa Charter' (WHO 1986), which defines five action areas for health promotion:

Build healthy public policy
Create supportive environments
Strengthen community action
Develop personal skills
Reorient health services

The model of health promotion presented in this chapter is entirely consistent with the Ottawa Charter, but has the advantage of setting out explicit categories of task for individuals, groups, and agencies to consider their scope as 'health promoters'.

WHO has also developed a number of health promotion initiatives, including a global programme on AIDS, a European programme on tobacco, the 'Healthy Cities' network, and, in partnership with the Council of Europe and the European Union, the European Network of Health Promoting Schools.

4.5.2 Health promotion and public health

Paralleling the growth in interest in health promotion in recent times has been a resurgence of interest in 'public health'. In the course of these developments, rhetoric has often been centred on 'the new public health', no doubt in the recognition of changes in public health challenges with the changing patterns of disease since the famous days of the turn-of-the-century Medical Officer of Health (MOH). This has not always been helpful: there has been a needless division of professional advocacy between health promotion and the new public health when in fact the advocates have generally been talking about the same sorts of measures.

Ideas as to what constitutes public health in the UK have been influenced greatly by the lasting impressions of the period 1948–74, when Medical Officers of Health, employed by local government, were concerned principally with prevention, while public hospital services came under the auspices of hospital boards.

An influential contribution to perceptions of public health was made in 1988, with the publication of 'Public Health in England' (the report of a committee of inquiry chaired by the Chief Medical Officer of the Department of Health, and hence eponymously known as the 'Acheson Report'; DHSS 1988). This document traced the history of public health in the UK and pointed out that immediately prior to 1948 almost all publicly funded preventive activities and health care were under the management of the MOH. It is apparently in returning to this spirit that the Acheson committee arrived at this definition of public health:

the science and art of preventing disease, prolonging life and promoting health through organised efforts of society.

Health promotion as defined in this chapter should thus be treated as a substantial and vital component of public health (Tannahill 1988*b*).

4.5.3 Health promotion and UK health strategies

A striking feature of the early 1990s has been a greatly increased emphasis on health promotion, set within the context of strategies for improving health. In Scotland, national policy statements *Health education in Scotland* (SOHHD 1991) and *Scotland's health: a challenge to us all* (Scottish Office 1992) have been followed by publications and initiatives in particular areas of concern, accompanied by an upsurge in investment in health promotion within the NHS and beyond, and a push towards building alliances for health (Anonymous 1993). England's *The health of the nation* strategy (Department of Health 1991, 1992*b*) has involved the setting up of working groups and task forces to address key health promotion issues, and has led to a wide range of activities and resources (Department of Health 1993), again with an emphasis on alliances. Parallel efforts have been mounted in Wales and Northern Ireland (Health Promotion Authority for Wales 1990; NIDHSS 1991).

Although the nations' strategies vary in detail, they have several things in common. They place health promotion at the top of the agenda of the NHS and other agencies; they highlight the need for everyone—national and local government, statutory and voluntary agencies, and communities—to work together to promote health; they identify priority topics—categories of health/ill-health and of behaviour—for action; and they set targets for achievement. The strategies have been criticized for what they have not said or achieved, but it should be recognized that they have provided fertile soil for the flourishing of health promotion in the UK, at all levels.

4.6 Assessing commitment

Reference has been made in the preceding section and in Chapter 3 to greatly increased attention to health promotion in recent times. How can we judge the extent to which rhetoric is matched by action? In this section, a framework is presented whereby the real level of commitment to health promotion in a given geographical location or organizational entity may be assessed under six interrelated headings: ethos, basic needs, policies, facilities, communication, and products (Fig. 4.5).

Fig. 4.5 Framework for assessing commitment to health promotion.

The framework arises naturally from the model of health promotion presented in Section 4.3, and pulls together the many strands of good practice from this and previous chapters. It is, in effect, a 'macro-audit' checklist, which may be adapted to be applied to a country, a city, a smaller settlement, an organization, etc. The items in the checklist may be tailored to the place or organization under scrutiny. In the account which follows, the framework is applied at the level of a country; the checklist questions used are illustrative, not exhaustive—ideally a full list would be developed as a result of public and professional debate. The reader may wish, using the same six headings, to devise a checklist for application to a city, smaller community, or other setting (for example, a workplace, school, or hospital). In considering the examples given below, it should be remembered that, just as local-level activity is facilitated by national action, international co-operation has an important bearing on what is achievable in a given country.

Ethos

There are four interlinking elements to look for: health strategies; commitment to reducing inequalities in health; interdisciplinary and interagency alliances; and community participation. Checklist questions include the following:

1. Is there a coherent national strategy for health, with health promotion at its heart?
2. Is a true commitment to reducing inequalities in health apparent from the strategy or otherwise?
3. Are there strong alliances for health at all levels? Do central government departments work together, and with other national agencies, on a health-orientated agenda? Are there appropriate, active alliances at regional, area, district, and locality levels? Is there adequate communication, collaboration, and coordination between levels?
4. Are there mechanisms for ensuring that members of the public are adequately informed about health issues, and that they can participate, at all levels, in identifying needs and opportunities for action, and in determining the action to be taken?

Basic needs

1. To what extent are basic needs satisfied with regard to: food, education, water and sanitation, housing, income, employment, and useful roles in society? What are the trends?
2. How equitable is the meeting of these needs? What are the trends?

Policies

1. Is improving health status a cardinal value in overall national and sub-national policy-making?
2. Is there a system whereby the actual or potential health consequences of national policy-making in all areas (not just 'health', but also, for example, housing, transport, employment, industry, environmental control, education, agriculture, and food production) may be assessed? Do national policies across all areas reflect a will to co-ordinate and maximize efforts to enhance positive health and prevent ill-health?
3. To what extent does legislation promote health? For example, is there a ban on tobacco promotion? What are the laws regarding the sale of tobacco, alcohol, and other relevant products to minors,

and concerning smoking and the use of alcohol in public places? Are motor vehicle seat-belts compulsory? What about health and safety and 'environmentally friendly' legislation affecting industry and the community more generally? How well are the laws monitored and enforced?

4. Are there coherent and sustained fiscal policies on tobacco, alcohol, food, motor vehicles, etc.?

5. To what extent do the policies of public, private, and voluntary sector organizations and institutions compensate for gaps in legal controls? Are there tobacco, alcohol, drug, food, exercise, and stress management policies in such organizations and institutions? Is the health service playing an exemplar role?

Facilities

1. To what extent are health services geared, on the ground, to prevention and the enhancement of positive health? Are preventive facilities (such as immunization and cervical screening) available to those who may benefit from them? What about the quality of the facilities provided? Are communication aspects of such services adequate? Is sufficient attention paid to the need to avoid unnecessary damage to well-being in the pursuit of health gain through prevention? Are population perspectives sufficiently taken into account in planning and delivering services?

2. To what extent are there amenities for the promotion of positive health? For example, does the population have good access to high quality indoor sports facilities, operated in such a way as to reflect a commitment to health promotion more widely (visible through, for example, health education; policies on smoking, drinking, and eating on premises; encouragement of people of all levels of ability, not just a sporting élite; and measures to reduce the risks of injury)? Do communities have sufficient access to safe routes for walking, jogging, or cycling—is motor traffic control sufficient, are there special, well-lit, and secure paths, etc?

Communication

1. Are there planned, comprehensive, and co-ordinated health education efforts through mass media and in settings and sectors (schools, the health service, the workplace, the voluntary sector, and other community settings)?

2. Do professionals and agencies, not just in the health service, fulfil their potentials for informing, motivating, and supporting people to attain and maintain good health? Do health professionals set an appropriate

example? Is there communication between members of the public on health promotion issues?

3. Are there open channels of communication to policy-makers, such that they are properly informed by relevant professionals and agencies, and by the public? Is the rationale for policy-making transparent?

Products

1. To what extent is safety taken into account in the design and promotion of a range of products, such as motor vehicles and household equipment?

2. Do people have ready access to health-promoting products? Are healthy choices made easier (for example, by clear product information, differential pricing or availability of health-promoting and health-damaging products)?

3. What trends are there in the consumption of products linked to ill-health (such as cigarettes, alcoholic beverages, and illicit drugs) and that of goods advocated through health education (for example, low-fat milk, fruit and vegetables, cycle helmets, and exercise clothes)?

The framework serves to illustrate the extent to which health promotion, if truly placed at the top of the national agenda, must permeate all aspects of society. Even the illustrative list of checklist items given above is a daunting one, which runs the risk of inducing paralysis rather than galvanizing action. The important principle is to build in from the start, in any geographical location or organization, the health promotion ethos. If this is done, the other things will follow, and sustained, substantial change will be more likely to be achieved than through the adoption of a piecemeal 'tinkering at the edges' approach to health promotion.

4.7 Conclusions

1. The customary classification of prevention as 'primary', 'secondary', and 'tertiary' is unsatisfactory.

2. Instead, four foci for prevention may be described, these accommodating notions beyond the mere prevention of disease.

3. Health protection is important in the promotion of positive health and in the prevention of ill-health. Strong action, however, is hampered by powerful vested interests.

4. 'Health promotion' is a highly fashionable term which has, unfortunately, been used in many different ways, often without clarification of meaning.

5. It is helpful, for the purposes of definition, planning, and action, to view health promotion as comprising efforts to enhance positive health and reduce the risk of ill-health, through the overlapping spheres of health education, prevention, and health protection. Empowerment is a cardinal principle of health promotion.
6. Health promotion programmes are best planned according to 'arenas' for health promotion, rather than health or behavioural topics.
7. Health promotion is a major and integral component of the World Health Organization 'Health for All' strategy and of the field of public health.
8. In the UK there has been a striking increase in emphasis on health promotion, set within strategies for improving health. This provides tremendous opportunities for development at all levels.
9. The level of commitment to health promotion in a geographical location or organizational entity may be assessed under six interrelated headings: ethos, basic needs, policies, facilities, communication, and products. Ethos is the most important of these.

5 Evaluation

In the previous two chapters we have presented models of health education and health promotion. These models delineate and define our subject area and thereby enable us to identify the activities with which we are legitimately concerned. This is only a start, however. There is a degree of concern both among health promotion specialists and within other professional groups that practice has advanced in a non-rigorous manner, and that the development and implementation of effective health promotion in the future depends on an emphasis being placed on sound health promotion evaluation now. Whilst this is widely accepted, there is often expressed also the caveat that the evaluation must be appropriate to health promotion, with respect both to its aims and objectives, and to its underlying ethos or ways of working. Given the variety of approaches integral to health promotion practice, a correspondingly wide range of evaluation methodologies (both qualitative and quantitative) is required. Moreover, given the creative and developmental nature of health promotion initiatives, a focus on outcomes only will lead to the loss of opportunities to learn lessons about approaches.

Evaluation is concerned with making judgements about the value of activities, and the collection of data (whether qualitative or quantitative) contributes greatly to our ability to make such judgements. We would argue, however, that good judgements depend not only on looking at data concerned with the process or outcomes of the initiative of interest, but also on relating this narrow perspective to an overall framework which incorporates an assessment of health need and a coherent health strategy for addressing that need. These points will be explored further within this chapter. Our concern is not with the 'how-to-do' of evaluation. Rather we aim to clarify why we need to evaluate health promotion activities and to examine some of the fundamental issues, whilst alerting the reader to the complexities involved.

5.1 What is evaluation?

Two slightly different views of evaluation pervade the literature on health promotion. From the first viewpoint, evaluation involves assessing an activity in terms of the aims or specific objectives of that activity. For example, Williams (1987; p. 81) has written as follows:

> . . . the purpose of evaluation is that it should demonstrate whether an activity has been successful or to what degree it has failed to achieve some stated aims.

Before we can evaluate, then, we need to be clear about the aims of the activity. We can then judge the value of the activity in relation to the degree of attainment of these aims.

From the second viewpoint, evaluation is a broader process. It involves assessing an activity by measuring it against a standard which is not necessarily related to the specific objectives or purpose of the activity. This approach has been advocated by Green *et al.* (1980; p. 123):

> We define evaluation simply as the comparison of an object of interest against a standard of acceptability.

Clearly, as in the first definition, the 'standard of acceptability' may refer to the achievement of aims or objectives. However, this is only one possibility. From this second viewpoint, evaluation may involve assessing an activity according to, for example, the ethics of the approach, the cost of the activity, or the reactions of the recipients or participants.

The first viewpoint may be viewed as a subset of the second. This latter viewpoint is helpful in a number of ways.

First, it is consistent with the fact that we are interested in answering not only the question 'Is the activity effective?', but also questions such as 'At what cost?', 'Using what means?', and 'With what consequences?' In other words, it is a reminder that we cannot be content only with showing that activities are effective at achieving the desired outcome.

Secondly, it clarifies the fact that we should assess the *processes* of health promotion as well as the *outcomes*. When the word 'aims' is used, it is often taken to imply some end-point or goal, and thus has limited and specific connotations. In the following section we advocate a broad interpretation of the term 'aims', to incorporate not only outcomes but also the various procedural aims of health promotion.

Thirdly, it leads us away from a narrow view of suitable outcome measures by alerting us to the presence of a range of standards of acceptability. It follows that a variety of assessment procedures may be appropriately employed in evaluation. The benefits of this are explored in Sections 5.3 and 5.6.

There are some advantages, then, in seeing evaluation in broad terms. Nevertheless, the evaluation activity must have its own clear aims, which are often worded as hypotheses to be tested, or research questions to be answered. Without such a focus, the resources invested in evaluation will not enable judgements to be made about value. Moreover, evaluation must always be relevant to the aims or objectives of the activity being appraised, and the measurements made need to be varied and appropriate. In Sections 5.3 and 5.5.8 we describe some of the types of measure which may be employed in evaluation. First, however, the terminology will be examined.

5.2 Definition of terms

Whilst there is a general consensus about the way in which many terms are used in discussions of the evaluation of health promotion activities, there seems to be some inconsistency concerning their specific meanings. Our purpose here is to clarify the meanings we attach to them.

The first term which requires definition is *aims*. As in everyday parlance, this term refers to the intention or purpose of an activity. There are three important points to be made about aims:

1. Aims are the planned, or derived, effects of an activity. They comprise a general statement of intent.
2. Aims tend to be broad, and may be broken down into specific *objectives*, each of which contributes in some way to its associated aim. Any one aim might generate a large number of objectives.
3. Aims may concern the long- or short-term consequences of a programme, or may refer to some aspect of the process of project or programme implementation or operation.

This final point requires some clarification.

Activities in the field of health promotion may be examined in three broad stages. The initial stage involves planning and design; the second, the 'running' (implementation and maintenance) of the initiative; and the third, observing the effects (both short- and long-term). Approaches to evaluation can, similarly, be described in relation to these three stages.

One of the reasons for evaluation is to enable improvements in design, either prior to the implementation of a new activity (through pre-testing) or with respect to the future introduction of similar initiatives (through ensuring the presence of a feedback loop linking evaluation findings to future plans). *Pre-testing* is important to ensure that health promotion messages and projects are tailored to their particular, defined, target group(s). In this respect, it is essential to pay attention to characteristics of the target group as well as to the language, design, and communication medium of the proposed project. Issues of importance in pre-testing include: relevance of the message, imagery, and communication media at personal and group levels; recall and comprehension of the message; credibility; appeal; quality; importance (whether it is worth paying attention and remembering the message); and the extent to which there is anything confusing, conflicting, or contradictory in the message or associated imagery. A useful discussion of pre-testing, together with a description of the techniques and instruments used in the process, is presented by Tones and Tilford (1994). The nature of the enquiry is such that qualitative methods using 'focus groups' (drawn from the target groups) are appropriate. Although the principles involved owe much to the disciplines of marketing and advertising, they are relevant to the full spectrum of methodologies employed by health promotion specialists and should be used more widely than in relation simply to mass media campaigns.

Evaluation also is of considerable importance with respect to informing the design of future initiatives. The main point here is that an integral part of programme planning must be a review of previous similar initiatives, in order that the lessons learnt through their evaluations can be incorporated into the design of the new programme. Without attention to this basic principle of good practice there is a risk of continually reinventing the wheel. In this respect, the issue of *replicability* is of particular relevance, and therefore an analysis of the component parts of an initiative is of paramount interest (see also Section 5.6.2).

The implementation and maintenance of an initiative are together referred to as the *process*. This second stage involves all the workings of the initiative, its different components, and their interactions. Clearly, this machinery has to be in order before any activity can be expected to work as planned. Evaluation of process is an essential step towards achieving the desired effects from an intervention.

The effects, or consequences, of an activity may be observed (if they exist) at any stage over a period of time after exposure to, or implementation of, the activity. For convenience we may distinguish between those consequences observed more or less immediately and those resulting after a longer period of time. Henceforth we shall refer to the former as *impact* and to the latter as *outcome*.

Commonly a simple distinction is made between *process evaluation* and *outcome evaluation*. Nutbeam *et al.* (1990) present a developmental model for the evaluation of health education programmes, which suggests that at the early stages of programme development, outcome evaluation should be dominant (to determine whether or not the desired endpoints are being achieved). Process evaluation then takes on greater importance at later stages of development, with the evaluation focusing on the potential for replicability of the programme. Whilst presenting this sequential relationship, the model does also clearly indicate that at most stages both process and outcome evaluation are relevant. Our view is that a simple dichotomy is unhelpful. There can be no consistent distinction drawn between measures of process and measures of outcome. Indicators which may be measures of process in one situation may be measures of outcome in another.

In evaluating a developed programme, we may be interested in any or all of the three facets—process, impact, and outcome—and we need measures of each. Collectively these can be termed *output measures*. In this sense, output refers to manufacture as well as yield, as it includes aspects of the programme process as well as the effects. This clearly differs from common epidemiological interpretations of the term, as for example: 'The immediate result of professional or institutional health care activities, usually expressed as units of service, e.g. patient hospital days, outpatient visits, laboratory tests performed' (Last 1988).

To summarize, the evaluation of an activity involves assessing it in relation to its aims or its (more specific) objectives. The aims and objectives refer to the intentions for the activity, both in terms of the way in which it operates or runs, and also in terms of its short- and long-term effects. These concerns—the subjects of the aims and objectives—are commonly referred to, respectively, as process, impact, and outcome. Together they constitute output. There are many measures of output which are relevant in the evaluation of health promotion initiatives. These are outlined in the following section.

5.3 Measures of output

The previous discussions have emphasized that evaluation must always be relevant to the aims and objectives of the activity being assessed, and these should be explicitly stated. It follows that the output measures (measurements of the process, of the immediate impact of activities, and of the long-term outcome) must also be appropriate to the aims and objectives. Measurements of individual behaviour will not always do. For example, sometimes the interest lies with economic measures, or educational measures, or assessment of change in social attitudes or in environmental conditions. We thus need a variety of appropriate measures of output.

In addition to being appropriate, the measures must meet the criteria of repeatability and validity. *Repeatability* refers to the extent to which a measurement gives the same answer when the subject is re-examined. Provided that there is no relevant change in the subject or conditions of assessment, a repeatable measure will yield consistent responses every time it is applied. *Validity* refers to the extent to which a measurement actually does measure what it purports to measure. The validity of a measurement may be tested by comparing it with another, accepted measure.

Figure 5.1 indicates a broad aim for health promotion (derived from Chapter 2), some of the associated objectives, and output measures which could appropriately be used in the evaluation of activities. Clearly, each measure has its own relatively specific use. Health promotion involves a wide range of diverse activities, and its evaluation is problematic for the many reasons described in Section 5.5, but there is a range of output measures and methods which can appropriately be used to evaluate the effects of activities.

Aim	Measures
To prevent ill-health while promoting positive health	Health indicators
	Measures of health status
	Quality of life scales

Objectives	Measures/Methods
To change knowledge and beliefs	Health knowledge
	Perceived risks
To change attitudes and values (inc. self-awareness & self-esteem)	Values-clarification
	Attitude scales
	Self-esteem scales*
To enhance decision-making skills	Assessment of behaviour
To change behaviour	Assessment of behaviour
To establish health-promoting environments	Environmental monitoring
	Policies in public places
To achieve healthful social change	Surveys of social attitudes/values
To foster empowerment of individuals and communities	Locus of control (e.g. MHLC scales**)
	Assessment of behaviour
To achieve the above in optimal and acceptable ways	Efficiency
	Cost effectiveness/cost benefit ratio
	Ethical assessment

*e.g. Rosenberg (1965); Coopersmith (1967); Lawrence (1981)
** Wallston and Wallston (1978)

Figure 5.1 A guide to health promotion evaluation.

The list in this figure is not wholly comprehensive but highlights those measures which are most frequently used. It is beyond the scope of this discussion to examine each in turn so we shall concentrate on some general points in relation to the measurement of positive health and ill-health.

Levels of health in individuals and in populations have conventionally been measured using *objective* indices, such as biochemical, microbiological, and radiological tests, blood pressure measurement, and behavioural assessment, in the first instance; and mortality, morbidity, and service utilization (e.g. bed occupancy) rates, in the second. However, it has become noted increasingly that these measures are not appropriate measures of the *health* of individuals and populations, in the complete sense of health as described in Chapter 2. There are several reasons for this:

1. In general they are measures or specific markers of illness and disease, and make no contribution to the measurement of positive health.
2. They are principally measures of the physical component of health and neglect the important mental and social aspects.
3. They are based on professional assessments and professional opinions of the crucial components of health. They therefore take little or no account of lay perceptions of health and lay priorities for health.

These objective measurements have thus been found to give misleading impressions about health. For example, a decreasing mortality rate does not necessarily mean an increasingly healthy population, just as the absence of abnormality in biochemical or radiological tests does not mean that the individual being assessed is healthy. More sophisticated indices are required to measure health status.

Another, more conceptual, difficulty is that the most common approach adopted when measuring health status is to take health (however defined) as the baseline, and to measure deviations away from this state, thereby yielding measurements of ill-health rather than of health itself. The continued persistence of this approach, despite the now widespread acceptance of the inadequacies of a purely 'medical model' of health and the concomitant need for a holistic view of health, reflect the difficulties of developing a measure of positive health—a measure which will be relevant to the majority of the population who at any one time are not experiencing a substantial impairment to their health. Bowling (1991) argues that a positive conception of health is difficult to measure because of the lack of agreement over its definition, and that positive health is composed of distinct components that must be measured and interpreted separately. As outlined in Chapter 2, we would agree that health may be assessed in terms of a set of properties, attributes, or characteristics. It is this conceptualization of health that has underpinned the work of many researchers involved in developing *subjective* indicators of health. This 'characteristics' approach is consistent with the various other models of health: it includes the perspective of social health; it incorporates the medical model of health as the absence of disease; and it emphasizes the experiental concept of feeling ill (or well), whether or not disease is present. In our view, this is the most useful way in which to view health, and it has practical relevance both for the measurement of health and for the implementation of health promotion activities relevant to the needs of particular target groups.

There are two broad types of health indicator: the health profile and the health index.

Health profiles provide a descriptive account of different aspects of health (such as pain, physical mobility, social life, etc.). Each of these aspects is described in quantitative terms, but the disparate measurements are not aggregated. Thereby a profile quantifying different aspects of health is yielded. The Nottingham Health Profile is a good example (see Hunt *et al.* 1986).

Health indices go a step further than the profiles, by aggregating measurements of many different aspects of performance and experience into a single value. For example, the McMaster Health Index Questionnaire (Chambers *et al.* 1976) is a measure of physical, social, and emotional functioning. There are 59 items in the questionnaire (split between physical function items, social function items, and emotional function items), and on each a score of 1 is given to a 'good function' response and a score of 0 to a 'poor function' response. The scores across all items are then totalled to produce an index of health. Another index of health, the General Health Questionnaire (GHQ) (Goldberg 1978) concentrates on broad components of psychiatric morbidity. It has several versions, ranging from the original 60-item format to the shortest 12-item version. Item scores are totalled to form the overall GHQ, and threshold levels are specified as definitions of 'caseness'.

Another type of single global indicator which has been developed and widely acknowledged is the 'Quality-adjusted life year' or QALY. QALYs may be used to combine quality and duration of survival in the assessment of programmes or services. This is more sensitive than the traditional measure of 'life expectancy', since acknowledgement is made of the fact that some activities may improve the quality of life whilst having no effect on its duration, and others may prolong life but have a detrimental effect on its quality (Williams 1983). QALYs have been most widely used by health economists and those interested in comparing different health care services. They are useful tools for decisions about the allocation of resources, but reservations have been expressed not only about the methodology of their derivation but also concerning their use as an 'automatic decision-making device' replacing political discussion and management judgements (Smith 1987).

Clearly the choice of which health indicator to employ will depend on the purpose for which it is being used. Within the field of health promotion, however, the profile approach is seen to have several advantages over the global health index.

First, the aggregation of different components into a single index inevitably results in the loss of information. Given the range of objectives of health promotion activities, it follows that the output measures should involve assessments of the various components of health rather than the reduction of information to a single value. This approach is also in line with our recommended conceptualization of health as a set of characteristics.

Secondly, whilst the development of a valid and reliable health profile is far from straightforward, it avoids many of the methodological difficulties inherent in the construction of indices, such as the problem of combining like with unlike, and of making assumptions about the extent to which some factors inevitably add more to the state of health than do others.

Thirdly, whereas the index approach is most useful for the assessment of outcomes of different interventions, or for comparing the effects of different health care services, health profiles provide more appropriate measures of the state of health of individuals and populations. They too can be used to compare the relative situations of individuals or groups, but this is not their sole purpose. The needs of health promotion, similarly, are more often concerned with detailed assessment of the state of health within a population of interest than with comparing this population to another.

Health authorities/boards have been charged with the responsibility of assessing the health needs of their resident populations. Much of the work carried out in this regard to date has focused on needs for health care, usually in relation to a particular specialty or set of conditions, and has thereby failed to incorporate lay definitions of health and to identify health needs that cannot be addressed through the provision of health services. There is currently, however, considerable interest in the assessment of needs of local communities, defined in relation to geographical localities. This shift in approach brings with it a shift in thinking, towards methodologies which involve local people, recognize the legitimacy of experiential and subjective perspectives, and endorse a broad conceptualization of health and its determinants.

A final distinction to be drawn in this analysis of health indicators is between those measures based on subjective perceptions (judgements made by the person whose health is being measured) and those based on an objective assessment, usually by a health professional. Although objective measurements are commonly of the index type, the subjective/objective distinction does not exactly correspond to the profile/index dichotomy. Historically, objective measures have been preferred as they have been viewed as more valid, being made by those with expertise in 'health', and more reliable, because they use techniques which measure something absolute, and are not dependent on someone's belief and opinion. These assumptions have now all been questioned, and subjective measures such as the Nottingham Health Profile have been found to be valid, repeatable, and, for our purposes, more appropriate measures of health.

There are several reasons why subjective indicators are of value to those involved with health promotion activities.

1. It is *perceived*, not necessarily *actual* situations which result in the adoption of health-related behaviours, including the demand for health care. For example, people who are dependent on alcohol may make artificial assessments of their position and of the effects of their drinking habits. As long as they do not perceive the existence of a problem they will not seek help, whether or not an objective assessment of their physical, mental, and social health indicates that they are in a poor state. The subjective indicator of health is a better predictor of behaviour than is the objective measure.
2. Because health promotion involves two-way communication and a 'bottom-up' approach, it is crucial for workers to be aware of, and to understand, the health beliefs and perceptions of the subjects with whom they are working. Only then can programmes be made appropriate and relevant to perceived needs. Moreover, activities which recognize lay beliefs will be more effective as they can tackle issues which are perceived as 'real', in a language known to their clients.
3. Subjective indicators are not restricted by professionally defined scales or terminologies. Instead they are based upon lay people's own assessments and personal valuation systems. This is clearly more

appropriate for health promotion, which looks beyond the medical model of health and is aiming to affect lay beliefs about health.

Subjective assessments of health are consistent with the overall philosophy of health promotion and they are not restricted by any one professional model of health. They are good predictors of behaviour, and provide an essential foundation for effective planning and communication about health-related issues.

5.4 Why evaluate?

There are five main reasons for evaluating health promotion activities. These are presented here, not in any particular order of importance. Different reasons will carry special relevance in different situations.

1. *To assess the extent to which projects are achieving their stated objectives.* Without evaluation we cannot know what effects specific initiatives have had. Have they had any effect either during implementation, or in the short- or longer-term post-implementation? If so, has the effect been positive, and in line with the desired objectives? This information is particularly important given the rapid rate of development of health promotion theory and practice. Changing circumstances, and the amount of innovative practice being delivered, mean that knowledge of approaches that have achieved favourable effects in the past may often be an inadequate basis for current decisions about practice. Evaluation is required to ensure the ongoing delivery of effective projects in current circumstances.
2. *To inform the development of materials and methods.* Projects may be having a desirable effect (or at least not a detrimental effect), but often they could be doing better. Stated objectives might be being met, but by sub-optimal means. Without evaluation we cannot compare different approaches or assess new refinements in methodology. The issues of interest here include a concern with effectiveness, but crucially also involve factors such as client/community views of relevance and acceptability, and economic concerns such as value for money.
3. *To ensure ethical practice.* By definition, health promotion activities aim to affect people's lives in a health-enhancing manner. In so doing they may cause inconvenience, discomfort, fear, or pain. Are the effects in terms of health gain justifiable? Do the outcomes of health promotion action warrant the personal expense, time, and intrusion into people's lives which they may incur? Do health promotion

projects use person-respecting methods? To what extent do they impair people's freedom of choice? Do they unjustifiably invade people's privacy? To what extent do they actually cause harm? Only by evaluating can we assess the costs and benefits of activities and thereby judge whether the effects of a particular approach are justifiable.

4. *To optimize use of resources*. Without evaluation we cannot tell whether health promotion activities deliver value for money. Of interest here is not only the need to optimize use of resources by prioritizing projects and programmes within an allocated health promotion budget, but also the broader strategic issue concerning the balance of investment between health promotion and other health services. In this context, the use of evaluation methods which enable health promotion to be compared with other services is crucial. Clearly, cost cutting must not be the only criterion of success. If it were, then the most successful initiatives would be those ensuring the death of people once they reached pensionable age (see p. 54). On the other hand, health service managers are accountable for the resources used, and must therefore always take value for money into consideration when making decisions about resource allocation.

5. *To assess the place of health promotion within overall efforts to achieve health gain*. Moving now beyond the evaluation of specific health promotion projects, there is a need to evaluate the contributions being made by programmes of health promotion more generally. Although there is fairly widespread acknowledgement that health promotion is 'a good thing', there exists alongside this a degree of scepticism about its processes and their effectiveness. Increased rigour is required within the health promotion profession to establish its credibility, and to ensure that its contributions are assessed appropriately within the context of an overall framework or strategy for the achievement of health gain at national and local levels.

For all these reasons it is important to evaluate health promotion projects and programmes. Once again, though, there should be a word or two of caution. Evaluation itself costs money: this is especially significant given the chronic underfunding of health promotion initiatives. Moreover, evaluation too may intrude into people's lives and cost them time and effort; it may involve them in the completion of questionnaires, which may be time-consuming and stressful, and in the provision of information which may be sensitive or personal. Often there is no feedback to these participants, and if there is it may be meaningless or incomprehensible to them. Is the inconvenience of the evaluation procedure justifiable?

These difficulties can be dealt with and remedied to a certain extent, and they certainly do not undermine the many advantages that may accrue from evaluation studies. The point is simply that just as health promotion activities should not be carried out at any cost, neither should evaluation be carried out at any cost.

An additional difficulty arises when we consider *who* it is that should be evaluating health promotion. There are four main categories of personnel most likely to be involved: academic or research institutions; commercial research organizations (including freelance researchers); health promotion specialists themselves; and other health authority staff, including health economists and public health specialists. There is, therefore, not a shortage of potential health promotion evaluators—if one has the money to pay for commercial services, or the availability locally of health authority or academic researchers for whom health promotion evaluation is a legitimate (or even a priority) activity. In practice however, much of the pressure to evaluate lands on the health promotion specialists themselves. Aside from the issue of objectivity (see Section 5.5.3), the fundamental difficulty here is one of skills and experience. Most health promotion specialists are recruited on the basis of their skills in delivering health promotion initiatives and most health promotion training relates similarly to these skills and the associated knowledge base. Without an increased investment in staff with the skills and the responsibility for evaluation within health promotion units, the specialism will be unable to respond to the need for increased rigour in its practice.

5.5 Issues in evaluation

The evaluation of health promotion initiatives is far from straightforward. Indeed there are difficulties to be encountered at all stages of the evaluation process, from its planning through its execution to the final stage of making recommendations. Two valuable papers (Green 1977; Baric 1980) have discussed difficulties relating to the evaluation of health education. These are, of course, of central relevance to the larger field of health promotion, and so the following discussion incorporates many of the issues identified by those two authors.

5.5.1 The difficulty of isolating the effects of a specific health promotion initiative

Within the field of health promotion there is often a variety of initiatives involving the same community, which aim to influence the same health factors and achieve the same health-enhancing change. These initiatives will include those delivered directly by local and national health promotion agencies, but also activities carried out formally and informally by other professionals and groups. In addition, all communities are influenced by background factors including legislation and policies, media features, and news items which are relevant to health issues, and which may or may not influence health factors in the same direction as the proactive health promotion activity. The problem, then, is to isolate the effects resulting specifically from one of these initiatives. Similarly, in observing a trend in a given index it is problematical to relate this with certainty to a particular health promotion input. For example, in the UK we have been observing a decline over the last forty years in the prevalence of cigarette smoking in the adult male population. How can we assess the relative contributions of health education, personal cessation supports (for example nicotine patches), and legislative and fiscal measures to this trend?

5.5.2 The need for acceptance of a wide range of evaluation methodologies

It follows from our broad interpretation of the evaluation process—as the assessment of activities in a variety of ways against a variety of standards—that a range of approaches to evaluation should be adopted. A great many theoretical frameworks, drawn from both the biomedical and the social sciences, have considerable relevance to the analysis and development of health promotion; and both qualitative and quantitative approaches to evaluation should be applied. The tendency to strait-jacket health promotion into models of biomedical evaluation focusing on outcomes ignores the creative, developmental components of health promotion and leads to a loss of opportunities to learn about approaches.

If it is accepted that many disciplines would usefully be involved in health promotion evaluation, then workers from a variety of backgrounds may take part in the process. There is thus a problem of integrating the range of expertise and the various approaches which arise from this multidisciplinary activity. There has, however, been some progress towards the integration of different approaches. Everly *et al.* (1987), for example, have examined ways of integrating behavioural and financial models in the evaluation of health promotion programmes in the workplace, to answer simultaneously the two questions, 'Does the programme work?' and 'At what cost?'

A necessary step towards integrating approaches is the acceptance of standardized procedures and terminology for evaluation. Green and Lewis (1987) have proposed standardization of this type for the evaluation of health education. However, we are a long way from having standard, accepted terminology and procedures for evaluation within and across all the domains of health promotion—and this acts as a barrier to effective and appropriate evaluation.

5.5.3 The issue of who should carry out the evaluation

In Section 5.4, we identified four broad categories of people who are involved in health promotion evaluation, and drew attention to the limited investment currently being made to ensure that within health promotion units there are staff with the skills and responsibility for monitoring and evaluating activities. Some issues need to be highlighted, however, if the health promotion specialist is to be seen as having a central role in evaluation. First is the issue of objectivity. Health promotion specialists' personal involvement with the service being evaluated may well bring with it subjective bias and preconceived ideas about its value. This needs to be recognized, and a division made, where possible, between practice and evaluation. Secondly, health promotion specialists, by the nature of their work, are usually driven by a strongly-held ideology. In this, they are not of course unique. Health economists are driven by a particular perspective, as are sociologists, public health medicine specialists, and so on. The issue here is to ensure that the assumptions, or ideology, underpinning a particular research approach or analysis are made explicit. Finally, the strengths of involving health promotion specialists in the evaluation of their discipline also must be recognized. They have a good understanding of the issues involved in health promotion practice, and therefore are likely to avoid the naïve assumptions made by some outside researchers. Moreover, involvement of practitioners in evaluation is the most likely route by which increased rigour will become integral to practice, and evaluation findings translated into action.

5.5.4 The need to evaluate health promotion in its entirety

In evaluating health promotion activities it is essential that we avoid focusing only on those issues that can be readily evaluated, to the neglect of the underpinning health promotion values and ethos. Health promotion is more than a set of definable projects, with their own specific objectives. Health promotion as a whole aims to achieve broader cultural and societal changes, within organizations, communities, and the population as a whole. In achieving this it depends critically on the involvement of other agencies. Efforts to evaluate health promotion programmes at this level (through the Healthy Cities network, for example) are at an early stage, but this is an area of work requiring urgent attention and investment.

5.5.5 Evaluation must be appropriate to the stage of service development

Within the health (and other) services, health promotion is still at a relatively early stage of development. Evaluators must therefore be careful to avoid making demands inappropriate to the stage of service development, or else the results of evaluation will inevitably be discouraging. Once again we see the clear need for evaluation of *processes*, particularly in relation to the development of new initiatives. Only once health promotion services are properly primed can we realistically expect them to be effective at achieving the desired impact or outcome.

5.5.6 Absence of experimental conditions

Scientific experiments demand rigorous conditions, standardization of environments, and precision of procedure. For the evaluation of health promotion programmes working with communities, however, conditions such as these will not be present. Moreover, we should not insist on total experimental rigour in situations where it is not justified. Health promotion programmes should not be restricted by the demands of evaluators to 'carry out the original plan no matter what', but rather should be allowed to develop to their full potential, taking advantage of the expertise and initiative of those implementing them.

5.5.7 Time factors

There is a problem of when to evaluate, as the outcome of an activity will vary at different time periods after the intervention. Some effects of health promotion are immediate whilst others are slow in emerging. Some effects are transient and others longer lasting. In the absence of prohibitively expensive and time-consuming longitudinal studies, various time-related problems in evaluation have to be recognized. These have been described as 'the dilemma of long- vs. short-term evaluation', and categorized as follows (Green 1977):

1. *Delay of impact*. This occurs, for example, when a process of attitude change has to be undertaken before behaviour change can take place. If we evaluate too soon after the intervention, then the behaviour change will not be observed.
2. *Decay of impact*. In some cases the intervention will have a more or less immediate effect which decreases over time. If we evaluate too late we will not measure the immediate impact; and if we do observe an effect we cannot assume it to be permanent.
3. *Borrowing from the future*. Sometimes interventions merely hasten behavioural change, such as smoking cessation, which would have occurred anyway. This may, of course, have real benefits, but we have to be careful not to overestimate the effects of an intervention.
4. *Adjusting for secular trends*. If the objective of an intervention is to increase the prevalence of a variable, and if this variable is on the increase anyway and we fail to adjust for this, we shall overestimate the benefits of the intervention. If the general trend is a decline in the variable of interest, then the benefit of the intervention may be underestimated.
5. *Contrast effect*. This may occur when a programme is terminated prematurely, or when the subjects have expectations which are not fulfilled. A consequently embittered group of 'clients' may act in defiance of advice on behaviour, producing a 'backlash effect'. Evaluation during, or soon after the intervention would measure the benefits but not the contrasting backlash which occurred after termination of the activity.

5.5.8 Performance indicators for health promotion

These points highlight the need for specificity in the identification of appropriate performance measures for health promotion, which relate clearly to the stated objectives of activities. Use of long-term outcome indicators is often inappropriate, and identification of intermediate and indirect indicators is to be encouraged. To give an example, in a community-based heart disease prevention project, the outcome indicator would be heart disease morbidity and mortality; intermediate indicators would include smoking prevalence, dietary behaviour, etc.; and indirect indicators would embrace, for example, the level of health professionals' participation in project components.

Intermediate indicators are of particular importance in the following three situations (Tones and Tilford 1994):

1. *Where the link between an outcome and some precursor event has been established only tentatively, or on the basis of probability:* for example, the relationship between particular personality types and the onset of coronary heart disease (CHD). In this instance, the effectiveness of health promotion action to produce a shift away from aggressive stress-associated behaviour patterns should not be judged in terms of the incidence of myocardial infarction in the population.
2. *Where a synergy, or interaction, is required between different approaches before the desired outcome can be achieved:* for example, educational inputs often require accompanying policy changes in order for the desired health outcome to be achieved.
3. *Where there is a time lag between the completion of a project and the desired outcome:* for example, the delay that is inevitable between the implementation of a health education package in school and the opportunity to assess whether it has had an effect on behaviour after leaving school.

In practice, intermediate indicators are the most commonly used for monitoring the effects of health promotion action.

5.5.9 Limitations of evidence-based decision-making

Despite the need for greater attention to evaluation, and the considerable benefits to be gained from using evaluation results to influence action, health promotion planning and practice and decisions about resource allocation cannot—and should not—be based on empirical evidence alone. These decisions need also to take account of management directives (whether local or national) which specify our priority areas for action and often set numerical targets to be met. These directives may also reflect particular political ideologies, and can lead to difficulties in accommodating local priorities and circumstances. As well as management directives, the views of local communities and consumers should be influential in affecting decisions about health promotion. The importance of involving local communities and consumers is now well recognized, but the views of these groups deserve much more attention than they currently receive. These views can form an invaluable addition to empirical evidence, which is often partial or inconclusive. Even substantial and expensive evaluations have a tendency to raise more questions than they answer.

Most importantly, decisions about priorities and resource allocation should not be made without recourse to an overall strategy or framework. Such a strategy should make explicit the philosophy as well as the methodologies adopted in the identification of need and priorities. St Leger *et al.* (1992; p. 184) present the following list of ideologies which could underpin the purchasing of health services:

1. An approach to maximize the economic wealth of the nation. This implies concentrating resources on those who are economically active or soon to become economically active.
2. A Benthamite approach, i.e. utilitarianism. This would seek to maximize some health 'good' for the greatest number. Significant majorities might get short shrift.
3. A Marxist/Structuralist approach. This might concentrate on reducing differences in health experience between social groups, i.e. the so-called 'health inequalities'.
4. An equitable approach, i.e. fair shares for all. It is assumed that there is a working definition of fairness.
5. A self-interest approach. At governmental level, this might entail taking the course of action least likely to lose votes.

These approaches are philosophically and operationally incompatible, and some are certainly incompatible with the values that underpin health promotion. Nevertheless, it might be the case that within any one health authority/board different members of staff or different divisions would be found to be working on the basis of different approaches, unless the philosophy that underpins the organization's strategy as a whole is made explicit.

5.6 Approaches to evaluation

So far we have discussed the evaluation process only in general
terms, as if the term 'evaluation' itself is an adequate explanation
of what is being done. The process is much more complicated
than that, however, and any of a variety of approaches to
evaluation may be adopted. When interpreting evaluation studies
it is important to consider the following issues at least:

— *When* was the evaluation carried out?
— *What* was evaluated?
— *Why* was the evaluation carried out?
— *How* was the evaluation carried out?

5.6.1 When was the evaluation carried out?

Evaluation studies which are carried out while the programme
of interest is still happening are known as *formative* evaluations,
and those which take place after it is ended are called *summative*
evaluations. Clearly, as was illustrated by the seat-belt legislation
in the UK, attitudes and behaviour are often found to change
after a policy is established. Thus attitudes detected during a
formative evaluation might not correspond to those identified
by a summative evaluation. Nevertheless, formative evaluations
are widely used as the basis of ongoing monitoring of programme
implementation and can provide invaluable information to ensure
that an initiative responds appropriately to participants' needs and
requirements.

5.6.2 What was evaluated?

Approaches to evaluation may be classified according to the
particular aspect of the programme which is to be evaluated:
process, impact, or *outcome* (as defined earlier on p. 80). Health
promotion programmes are commonly evaluated in terms of
impact, using intermediate indicators. Evaluation of this type
is relatively easy and inexpensive to carry out; and it helps to
provide an answer to the question of whether the programme
'works' in the short term.

In addition to the evaluation of impact, we have argued for the
importance of process evaluation. Process evaluation permits an

analysis of the component features of a project, yielding detailed information of direct relevance to the development of materials and methods, and an understanding of the applicability and replicability of approaches to other settings.

Outcome evaluation addresses the question: 'Does it work in the long term?' It is important to distinguish between 'ultimate' outcome (in terms of health status) and other outcomes (such as cognitive or behavioural outcomes) more directly related to a programme's stated objectives. Health promotion as a whole needs to be seen to be contributing to 'ultimate' outcome, but measures with a more direct association to health promotion projects are the more appropriate for gauging the effects of an intervention. It is crucial to ensure that the conclusions drawn from an evaluation are appropriate to the 'level' of measure used.

5.6.3 Why was the evaluation carried out?

In Section 5.4 we listed five main reasons for evaluating health promotion activities. An understanding of the purpose of the evaluation is essential for the interpretation of evaluation results. The recipient of an evaluation report needs to know not only the aims and objectives of the initiative of interest, but also the aims and objectives of the evaluation study. Only with this understanding can the relevance and quality of the evaluation itself be judged—and this, of course, is a prerequisite to making any judgement about the value of the initiative of interest on the basis of its evaluation. The danger to be avoided is that of uncritical recipients of evaluation making planning or resource decisions based on poor quality evaluations.

Different approaches to evaluation need to be distinguished, and a useful classification is that presented by Arnold (1972). Building on his analysis, four types of evaluation can be identified.

1. *Evaluation of the complete system.* In this approach, interest lies above all in assessing the extent to which the programme is functional as a whole. The component parts are of interest with respect to how they interrelate and contribute to the aim of the total programme, but there is little interest in looking at specific projects in any detail.
2. *Evaluation of particular strategies.* The purpose of this type of evaluation is to gain an understanding of the relative effectiveness and ethical acceptability of particular approaches. Here the focus

is on appraising different approaches to practice, with an interest both in understanding the processes and in assessing value with respect to impact and outcome. This approach differs from the previous approach in that it does not apply a systems perspective, but rather focuses on only particular, identified, components of the system.

3. *Evaluation of programme management.* This approach seeks to understand how an initiative works in practice and then to relate this back to its proposed effectiveness at the planning stage. Evaluation with this model can assess the extent and effects of any changes that have occurred from planning to implementation. An understanding needs to be obtained not only of the changes that have occurred but also of the reasons for these changes.

4. *Relevance evaluation.* This type of evaluation appraises the extent to which initiatives are up-to-date and appropriate. One approach here is to appraise current practice critically in the light of current knowledge as presented in the literature. Alternatively, the relevance of the intiative can be assessed by seeking the views of participants, recipients, potential recipients, policy makers, and other interested parties. This approach is adopted particularly during pre-testing (see p. 79) and in formative evaluations, but its value more generally should not be ignored.

The rigorous development of the specialty of health promotion depends on quality evaluation of each of these types.

5.6.4 How was the evaluation carried out?

The decision about how to evaluate is often determined by the availability of resources, and by the feasibility of different evaluative designs. We have recognized the contributions to be made by many disciplines, and argued for a diversity of approaches. However, the close links between health promotion and public health have meant that the evaluation of health promotion programmes has traditionally owed much to epidemiological method. In these studies, various designs have been adopted.

Basic evaluation can be carried out simply by *record-keeping*. For example, routine data collected about attendance at outpatient clinics will indicate fluctuations which may be associated with relevant health promotion initiatives and provide an indication of their impact.

Simple evaluation by observing trends over time does not permit us to conclude whether these trends result from health promotion activities or whether they would have occurred anyway. One way of clarifying this is to make a comparison with a comparable location where the intervention of interest is absent. This is known as a controlled-comparison (*quasi-experimental*) approach. Another comparative design involves comparing the situation of interest with others where there is a similar intervention.

In the comparative designs described above, comparison groups fall outside the sphere of influence of the evaluation exercise. Another approach is to have an experimental design similar to that used in a clinical trial. This is a *controlled-experimental* approach. Subjects (or collections of subjects) are randomly assigned to an intervention group or a control group. A more complex approach along the same lines of design involves more than two groups, exposed to different 'doses' of intervention.

Clearly these experimental approaches have limited application for the evaluation of many health promotion initiatives. Some- times they would be unethical: how could we justify withholding education about health services, for example, from a group of the population? In other circumstances they might be infeasible: for instance, how could a group of the population be made exempt from legislative or fiscal measures? Moreover, except in certain specific circumstances, such as the use of preventive medication, the 'double-blind' ideal of the clinical trial cannot be achieved in health promotion evaluation: there is, for example, no placebo for a health education intervention. Thus, whilst this controlled-experimental design is the most desirable epidemiologically, its applicability to the evaluation of health promotion practice is limited.

The evaluation of health promotion programmes must be carried out in the field, in the arenas in which the programmes are taking place. We cannot expect to achieve laboratory conditions, and we should not expect to. This point is made clear by Green *et al.* (1980; p. 140):

The problem with the more complicated designs is that they usually have to be carried out under highly controlled conditions, which makes behavioural circumstances unusual or unnatural . . . what one gains in neutral validity through the more rigorous randomised procedures one may sacrifice in feasibility and generalizability of findings.

Often, the quasi-experimental approach will be found to be the most appropriate and acceptable epidemiological method.

5.7 Conclusions

1. We advocate a broad view of evaluation, involving a range of approaches and output measures.
2. Evaluation of health promotion activities must be relevant to the aims of these activities. Appropriate aims are diverse and include many objectives in addition to the traditional educational ones of changing beliefs, attitudes, and behaviour.
3. We have identified the main reasons for evaluating health promotion programmes. In summary, we need to ascertain the effects of programmes, assess the methods employed, and examine the use of resources.
4. It is essential not to expect from health promotion activities results inappropriate to the stage of service development. Over-ambitious demands will inevitably be frustrated. At early stages of development there should be strong emphasis on evaluating the *process* of health promotion.
5. The methodology employed for evaluation should not be so epidemiologically rigorous as to inhibit initiative and development in the field. The evaluation of health promotion programmes must be carried out in the arenas in which the programmes are taking place, and it is inappropriate to expect to achieve laboratory conditions.

6 Models in action

The purpose of this chapter is to demonstrate, through selected examples, how the various models presented so far may be translated into practice. We shall start by considering an actual case study in health *education*, to do with a topic-based response to an emergent health hazard (snuff-dipping products). We shall then look in some detail at the applicability of the model of health *promotion* (see Chapter 4), in turn, to a disease topic (coronary heart disease), a risk factor topic (alcohol), and two key arenas (primary health care and schools).

6.1 Health education and a risk factor topic

With reference to the model of health promotion (Fig. 6.1), this case study is an example of health education for preventive health protection (the domain labelled number 4 in the figure). That is to say, the initiative which will now be described represents an attempt to secure, through education, preventive regulatory action against a specific health hazard.

6.1.1 The problem

In Scotland, in 1985, health professionals, politicians, trades unionists, Action on Smoking and Health (ASH), the media, and parents of young children joined forces in protest against 'Skoal Bandits'. US Tobacco Inc. had opened a factory in East Kilbride to manufacture these products, little teabag-like sachets containing moist tobacco, designed to be placed in the mouth between cheek and gum (a practice known as 'snuff-dipping').

Disquiet about these and other snuff-dipping products (SDPs) centred mainly around the facts that they had been shown to contain known carcinogens (Harrison 1986), that they had been linked to cancer of the mouth in the United States (Winn *et al.* 1981; US NIH 1986), and that an expert committee had declared this association to be causal (DHSS 1985). In addition, snuff-dipping has been implicated in lesser mouth problems, such as recession of the gums. The problems are magnified by the likelihood of nicotine dependence, and widened out by the attendant possibility of 'graduation' to smoking.

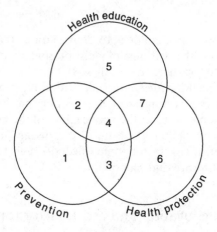

Fig. 6.1 The model of health promotion.

Concern was focused largely on young people: in the United States snuff-dipping had become very popular with youngsters, especially boys, encouraged by general product imagery (such as the masked bandit logo of Skoal Bandits and the association of SDPs with baseball heroes through advertising) and promotional ploys (including the giving out of free samples at rodeos). In the UK the style of promotion had disregarded the spirit of the voluntary agreement not to encourage the use of SDPs by young people.

A strong element of outrage was added to the public protest by reports that a government department had contributed around £1 million of public funds towards US Tobacco's East Kilbride venture (Cameron 1985). A tinge of farce was contributed by the fact that the Government's health departments were so concerned about snuff-dipping that letters were sent to all doctors and dentists warning them about the dangers of the practice and discouraging the use of the products.

This case study is concerned with the response to snuff-dipping in one English Health Region—East Anglia. In late 1985, following media coverage of the Scottish campaign against SDPs, the East Anglian Regional Health Promotion Group (EARHPG) set up a small task group to monitor the situation locally and devise action as appropriate. (EARHPG was a body set up by the Regional Health Authority but including representatives from various agencies outside the health service.) Over the next few months several low-key tasks were undertaken, including the provision of information to health and local authority officers, community health councils, and Members of Parliament throughout the region.

Action had to be stepped up in mid-1986, following reports that SDPs were being promoted and sold in East Anglia.

6.1.2 Options for action

EARHPG considered a proposal for a region-wide media campaign in support of a public petition for a national ban on SDPs. This was rejected. At the time there was much to suggest from official attitudes and actions that a ban would not be forthcoming: without this outcome the exercise might have backfired by stimulating interest in, and thus demand for, products which were as yet not widely available. The risk of inadvertent promotion of SDPs similarly ruled out other high-profile options (such as the production of an education package for schools).

Instead, a low-profile initiative, led by the Regional Health Promotion Officer, was decided upon. The principal aim of this was to discourage potential retailers from promoting or selling SDPs.

6.1.3 The retailers' initiative

The Regional Health Promotion Officer asked the 20 local authority environmental health departments in the region to provide names and addresses of potential retailers of SDPs. Each identified retail outlet was sent a locally produced leaflet which gave information about the products and their dangers, and outlined action already taken in the UK and abroad. An accompanying letter drew particular attention to the EARHPG's concern that children were especially vulnerable, and invited retailers to sign and return (by Freepost) a tear-off slip, thereby pledging not to promote or sell SDPs. The campaign was launched with a press release which emphasized the low-key nature of the project and stressed the need to avoid potentially counter-productive publicity.

A follow-up mailing of the campaign materials was undertaken some four months after the launch.

6.1.4 Results

Two thousand, four hundred potential retail outlets were successfully contacted. By the end of the campaign, 1309 signed pledges had been received (797 in the first phase, 512 in the second).

In addition, 'bottom-up' action by retailers resulted in eight major national/sub-national chains pledging not to promote or sell SDPs in any of their stores.

6.1.5 Discussion

The campaign represents an appropriate and effective response to a new health hazard. It is clearly preferable to block such hazards at source than to depend on public health education once they have become established. Furthermore, the campaign was successful in its important objective of avoiding unwanted publicity, thanks to good relationships with local media. Another notable feature was the fruitful collaboration between health service staff, local authority officers, and others.

The project demonstrates how, in the absence of strong national regulation, health education involving crucial power-holders can result in local preventive health protection measures and can directly stimulate action far beyond the locality in question. Also, it is to be hoped that a local initiative of this type, coupled with activities elsewhere, can contribute to a climate in which legislation is more likely. Certainly in 1990, following wide consultation, UK Health Ministers decided to ban SDPs under the Consumer Protection Act, 1987.

6.2 Health promotion and a disease topic

Not surprisingly, much effort has been devoted in the UK towards devising strategies for health promotion aimed at the prevention of coronary heart disease (CHD), the nation's largest single cause of death. We shall now use the health promotion model (Fig. 6.1) as a planning tool for CHD prevention, referring to the domains of activity as numbered in the figure.

1. Preventive activities relating to CHD include hypertension case-finding, the provision of nicotine-containing chewing gum to aid smoking cessation, and the effective management of predisposing conditions (such as diabetes mellitus and hypothyroidism).

    The role of mass blood cholesterol 'screening' has been the subject of considerable controversy in recent times. We shall not go into the opposing views in any depth here. We shall simply report that an expert panel has concluded that 'mass measurement of blood cholesterol levels in the population is not justified' (King Edward's Hospital Fund for London 1989). There is, however, a consensus in favour of blood cholesterol testing for selected individuals (such as people with a family history of 'premature' CHD, and people with known predisposing conditions).

2. This domain includes health education aimed at influencing lifestyle on the grounds of CHD prevention (important risk factors being smoking, certain aspects of diet, and lack of exercise), and that which encourages the uptake of any relevant preventive service (see domain 1 above).

3. Apposite preventive health protection measures would include those concerned with fundamental health determinants relevant to CHD (such as socio-economic disadvantage), and those aimed at specific risk factors (for example, fiscal action on tobacco—see p. 52, the control of tobacco advertising and promotion, and other policies on tobacco, food, and exercise in the workplace and elsewhere).

4. This includes educational efforts to secure appropriate preventive health protection measures (see domain 3 above).

    [We now come to consider the place of *positive* aspects of health promotion in relation to CHD, which are often neglected as a result of the essentially negative focus of preventive programmes.]

5. Both aspects of this domain of positive health education—that concerned with encouraging certain behaviours on positive health grounds, and that aimed at developing positive health attributes (see p. 60)—are highly relevant to the promotion of lifestyles which protect against CHD.

6. Similarly, the health protection measures for CHD prevention have additional positive benefits (for instance, policies on smoking positively improve the physical environment—see p. 60), and this should be reflected in the advocacy of such regulations and policies.

6.3 Health promotion and a risk factor topic

There is much concern over the growing problems associated with the use of alcohol. These include physical, mental, and social effects, not only on drinkers themselves but also on their families and society at large. Once again the health promotion model (Fig. 6.1) may be used to explore possibilities for action, as follows.

1. Preventive provision in this context would include measures designed to detect problem drinking or its deleterious effects as early as possible, and self-help groups and other agencies aimed at reducing the impact of alcohol problems.

2. Once again there is a place for preventive health education—to discourage situational, acute, or chronic misuse of alcohol on risk-reduction grounds, and to encourage the use of preventive services (see domain 1 above).

3. Preventive health protection would include fundamental aspects of public policy (in recognition of the links between social pressures and the use of drugs of solace). Specific legislation might address the sale of alcohol (for example, regulations concerning age or more general questions of accessibility to alcohol—for instance, through supermarkets), its advertising and promotion, or its consumption (for example in football grounds and other public places). The desirability of regular increases in duty has already been discussed (see p. 53). In recent times there has also been an upsurge of interest in devising and implementing workplace alcohol policies.

4. Once more, education is necessary to encourage preventive health protection.

5. Education concerning alcohol need not, and should not, be confined to *preventive* considerations. It is important (in schools, for example) to employ approaches to health education which encourage people to look at alcohol—its responsible and irresponsible use—in relation to subjective well-being and more objective measures of performance, rather than merely painting alcohol as 'a bad thing'. In doing this, we can try to stimulate a culture more favourable to the consumption of non-alcoholic and low-alcohol drinks. We can also promote ways of using leisure time other than by drinking. Moreover, as with the CHD example, the fostering of positive health attributes is of crucial relevance to alcohol. We should be developing and evaluating work on assertiveness and stress management training in relation to alcohol use, and we should be trying to foster self-esteem and nurture decision-making skills.

6. Likewise, positive objectives should be incorporated into alcohol-related health protection efforts. The use of alcohol-free and low-alcohol alternatives could be encouraged by regulations on differential pricing (comparable to those to do with unleaded petrol), and by policies favouring their promotion in an attractive manner (reinforcing the educational efforts outlined under domain 5 above). We could look at ways in which we could improve the environment of licensed

premises in such a way as to promote the responsible use of alcohol and the freedom (actual and perceived) to choose non-alcoholic drinks. Policies which lead to the provision of attractive and accessible leisure facilities as an alternative to bars would also be worthy of attention.

7. Health education efforts must be directed at securing measures of the sort described under domain 6 above.

6.4 Health promotion and an arena—primary health care

The examples presented as Sections 6.2 and 6.3 serve to illustrate that the health promotion model can be readily applied to diseases and risk factor topics. In the course of these illustrations, important areas of commonality in the area of positive health education will, however, have been noted (see also p. 44). Indeed, in considering health education in relation to CHD—both preventive and positive in orientation—we have seen that the aspects of lifestyle, lifeskills, and environment to be addressed are of great relevance to other aspects of (negative and positive) health. These observations in practical examples reinforce our earlier endorsement of planning and prioritizing health education and health promotion programmes in communities primarily according to *arenas* rather than *topics* (see p. 64).

In keeping with this advocacy, we shall conclude this chapter by considering health promotion in two arenas, starting with primary health care. The importance of health promotion in this setting is reflected in the UK in the 1990 contract for general medical practitioners (GPs) (Chisholm 1990), modified in 1993. The reader should bear in mind key principles of health education (pp. 36-9).

The account which follows focuses on the primary care team as commonly defined (GPs and immediate colleagues), but it should be noted that the roles of other primary care professionals, including general dental practitioners, community pharmacists, and optometrists, in health promotion may similarly be addressed (and indeed that the concept of the primary care team may be expanded to include such professionals).

1. The primary care team is involved in the provision of immunization and cervical screening. The UK GP Contract includes obligations with

regard to health assessments for new patients and for patients aged 75 and over. Under a banding system of remuneration for health promotion activities, it sets out qualifying requirements in relation to the collection of information on patients' smoking status, blood pressure, body mass index, alcohol consumption, family history, diet, and physical activity—all of which may be viewed as 'screening' in the widest sense. A great deal of interest in recent times has centred on whether health checks should be proactively and systematically offered to the general adult population through primary care. Taking into consideration evidence from randomized controlled trials (Family Heart Study Group 1994; ICRF OXCHECK Study Group 1994), the predominant view is that health assessments of patients aged 16–74 should be carried out opportunistically, with more proactive efforts in relation to this age group being reserved for those who have previously been identified as being at particular risk of preventable disease, and to reaching others who are most likely to be at risk. Further research evidence is awaited. As indicated in Section 6.2, there is now a consensus that whole population blood cholesterol screening is not appropriate and that cholesterol measurement should be confined to individuals identified as being at high risk of cardiovascular disease, as part of a broader process of risk assessment. It is generally accepted that routine urinalysis for glucose and protein is not warranted.

2. In communicating with their patients or clients about aspects of health, primary care professionals are inevitably engaged in health education. Viewed in this light, health education is not something into or out of which the primary care team can opt. Rather it is an integral part of practice. It is important to ensure that professionals' communication with their patients takes account of the principles presented in Section 3.5. Despite undeniable time constraints, primary care professionals can broaden out the focus beyond the subject of a given patient contact, to address major aspects of behaviour, including smoking, alcohol consumption, diet, exercise, and sexual behaviour. It has, for example, been demonstrated that the simple matter of advising someone to stop smoking may trigger cessation (Russell *et al.* 1979). Effectiveness can be enhanced—and time saved—by backing up verbal advice with appropriate educational materials. These should be concerned with the 'how to' of behavioural change and maintenance, not merely the 'what'. The primary care team also has an important part to play in promoting the uptake of preventive provision, including the relatively new breast screening service. In communication with their patients about such services (for example, about the implications of a suspicious or positive cervical smear), professionals should endeavour to ensure that health gain through prevention is not undermined by unnecessary reductions in well-being. Finally, there is a need for

piloting, with proper evaluation, of health education approaches such as group sessions and audiovisual materials (in, for example, health centre waiting rooms).

3. Health protection policies, such as non-smoking policies, can be created for primary care premises.

4. Members of the primary care team can play an active part, both as individuals and as groups (for example, through their own professional organizations or networks), in encouraging local and national policies to protect against ill-health. Primary care professionals have an important advocacy role, and indeed may view themselves as something akin to health MPs—'political' representatives of their practice lists in the face of threats to health, such as poor housing, unemployment, poverty, or dangerous industrial processes.

5. Health education in primary care must take on board the importance of positive health as a motivation for behaviour change. For too long health professionals have recommended alterations in lifestyles in an off-putting manner—reinforcing perceptions that a healthful lifestyle has to be dull, painful, self-sacrificing, or otherwise unpleasant—rather than painting positive images. Also, efforts must be made to use consultations and other contacts to help the development of the positive health attributes referred to repeatedly in this chapter and elsewhere. A very basic example of recognizing the importance of skills rather than simply information is to facilitate dietary modification by providing straightforward recipes instead of merely giving advice to reduce fats, increase fibre, and so on.

6. Health protection policies for the primary care setting will once again have positive aspects (for example, the clean air benefits of a non-smoking policy).

7. In fulfilling their potential role as health protection advocates, primary care professionals should remember also the positive quality of health protection measures beyond their premises (for instance, by pressing for decent local leisure facilities in the interests of positive health—well-being and fitness).

The repeated reference above to the primary care *team* is important. Proper teamwork requires a power balance distinct from that implicit in models of *delegation* from the doctor to others. It involves recognition and appropriate utilization of team members' skills, and the earning, and granting, of mutual professional respect. It will be clear from the above account that specific inputs on disease and risk factors are essential. We have never denied this (see p. 66). Our argument is simply that we need to develop programmes, in primary care and elsewhere, in a *co-ordinated* manner, bringing together the interlinking strands of preventive and positive health education in a participatory model of communication, and integrating education work with health protection efforts and with preventive activities such as screening. The challenge of co-ordination within a primary care team is a pressing one. We believe that every primary care team should have a nominated co-ordinator for health promotion, who should liaise with a health promotion specialist concerned either specifically with primary care throughout a health board area (or district), or with the various settings and groups in a particular community patch. The role of the co-ordinator would build on the strengths of the Oxford 'facilitator' model (Fullard *et al.* 1987), while taking into account the broad-based approach to health promotion espoused here.

6.5 Health promotion and an arena—schools

There are several reasons why the school is a key arena for health promotion. First, in accordance with a 'prevention is better than cure' philosophy, it is better to encourage young people to adopt healthful lifestyles than to try to change unhealthful behaviour patterns in adulthood. Secondly, there is evidence (notably in relation to CHD) that the risk factors for disease in adulthood often originate early in life. Thirdly, schools provide a unique opportunity to augment other influences on health-related behaviour with properly planned programmes of health education, whereby inputs in relevant subject areas, such as biology, home economics, and physical education, are co-ordinated with one another, and may be complemented by a programme of personal, social, and health education.

Our discussions so far in this chapter have taken a deliberately fragmented look at health promotion in order to illustrate the model fully. In this example we seek to examine health promotion less artificially and more cohesively, starting with a look at health education as a whole in the school setting.

6.5.1 Health education in schools

Traditionally, health education in schools was concerned with 'hygiene and cleanliness', with minimizing the risks of infection.

Partly as a result of the changing patterns of ill-health and largely due to recognition of the broader scope of health issues, the amount and breadth of health education in schools have increased greatly. Many of the changes can be linked to the ideas and models presented in earlier chapters.

Official recommendations have been made for a co-ordinated approach to health education in schools. Similar to our recommendations for primary care, the presence of a named co-ordinator in each school has been advocated.

Modern approaches to curriculum development in health education have emphasized the principle of the 'spiral curriculum', issues being dealt with in appropriate ways at appropriate ages. They have also taken a lifeskills approach, stressing concepts such as self-esteem, empowerment, and decision-making skills, rather than a purely information-based approach (Schools Council 1977*a*, *b*, 1982). This requires small-group teaching methods.

Schools offer an excellent opportunity for such labour-intensive efforts to educate for positive health simultaneously with attention to health hazards and available preventive services.

Research has shown school-based health education to be capable of producing positive effects on beliefs, attitudes, and behaviour, both short- and long-term. It has, however, been repeatedly found that the outcomes expected on the basis of previous evaluation are not necessarily achieved in practice. One reason for this is the conflicting messages presented to young people in schools: attention to self-empowerment may be at odds with pupils' lack of control over their lives at school; teaching about the benefits of good nutrition may clash with practical cookery classes or the food served in the canteen; advocacy of the need for health protection measures may fall in the face of smoking in the staff-room. The point is that even 'modern' approaches to health education in schools, comprehensively planned, are not enough on their own. The school as a whole must become a health-promoting environment, in terms of ethos, health protection policies, and provision of appropriate preventive services: health education in the formal curriculum must be matched by opportunities through the informal curriculum, and by a consonant 'hidden curriculum'. In short, health education in schools must take place within the overarching concept of the health-promoting school (SHEG and SCCC 1990; WHO, Council of Europe, and Commission of the European Communities 1993).

6.5.2 Preventive services and health protection

Health education may be supplemented by the provision of appropriate preventive services, such as rubella immunization and dental measures, within the school. Moreover, health education may be reinforced by the provision of a positively healthful and safe environment in the school through regulatory action, affecting teachers as well as pupils. An important aspect of health protection in schools would be to ensure that exercise facilities are seen as available to all pupils rather than only to the sporting élite: this would be expected to enhance self-esteem as well as physical fitness.

6.5.3 Beyond the school

Another potential reason for a lack of success in schools' health promotion is that of 'culture clash' between the school and the home and elsewhere. This can occur when values promoted at school conflict with mores in families, peer groups, and so on. It follows, then, that schools' health promotion must be linked to efforts to influence the broader social environment. Once again health promotion specialists have an important part to play.

6.6 Conclusions

1. The appearance of a new threat to health may warrant a specific, topic-based health education initiative aimed, for example, at securing health protection action. Where the new hazard is a product, the health education initiative may be best kept low-key in nature, to prevent the inadvertent stimulation of awareness of, and demand for, the harmful product.
2. The obtaining, through education, of local regulatory action may compensate for an absence of official control.
3. The model of health promotion presented in Chapter 4 may be used as a planning framework for action against a specific disease or risk factor. The model is, however, best used for the full exploration of health promotion opportunities in key arenas, leading to the development of integrated programmes tailored to the particular needs of these arenas.
4. Primary health care and schools are vitally important for integrated

programmes of health promotion. In both cases there is a pressing
need to tap the potential more fully.

Acknowledgement

We are grateful to Mrs Diane Fenner, formerly Regional Health
Promotion Officer, East Anglian Regional Health Authority, for
her kind permission to present the campaign against snuff-dipping
as a case study.

Part 2 Values

Introduction to Part 2

Some of our key concepts in Part 1 were modelled in terms of values—health in terms of well-being arising from the exercise of basic human qualities, and health education and promotion as processes which enhance that well-being. It is therefore helpful to think of the knowledge or technical base and the value or moral base of health promotion in terms of the analogy of a seamless garment. In discussing values we are simply turning the garment round and looking at the weaving from another angle.

We begin Part 2 with a discussion of the nature of attitudes and how they can be changed. Attitudes are perhaps the central concepts of the book because they are a focus for beliefs, feelings, and behaviour, and therefore express our values. Lasting changes to the health of a community must therefore come about through changes in attitudes, both personal and societal.

We consider in some detail what it is to value something, and what are the values which are essential to the flourishing of a society and an individual. These values we link via the idea of autonomy. But, since people are essentially social, autonomy is best expressed in the concept of citizenship. We repeat the point, which was stressed in Part 1, that autonomy is not something everyone in fact has—it is something to be achieved. To be a citizen, in the true sense, is to be *empowered*.

This conception does not fit easily with the traditional ideas of liberalism. In our view of health promotion, people should not see themselves as independent pursuers of their own interests; there is a communal good as well as individual goods—this is what is meant by calling people 'citizens'. Health promotion can be seen, from the perspective of Part 2, as an attempt to make this ideal of the citizen a reality. In particular, modifications of the liberal position arise in our conception of social justice.

Sometimes it is said that traditional medicine and health care are scientific and based on fact, whereas health promotion is moralistic; medicine deals with the 'is' and health promotion deals with the 'ought'. This view, which is generally intended as a criticism of health promotion, is confused. The truth is that *both* medicine *and* health promotion have a scientific basis, and *both* deal with prescriptions for improving the quality of life. The differences are between perspectives: the individual and the societal; the negative and the positive; the curative and the preventive; the reductivist and the holistic.

To say this is to say nothing necessarily disparaging of either; many of those in health care or health promotion can adopt either point of view as appropriate. Both points of view strive to be scientific, but neither is value-neutral. In this part of the book we try to express the scientifically based theory of health promotion in its value setting, which is nothing less than that of the good society—one which is conducive to the pursuit of 'a state of complete physical, mental, and social well-being'.

7 Attitudes, beliefs, and behaviour

Attitudes are often viewed as being central to health promotion. They affect the ways in which individuals, groups, and communities respond to health promotion initiatives; are linked to health-related beliefs and behaviours; and are directly and indirectly associated with health status. Also, as we shall see in Chapter 9, our values can be regarded as a subset of our attitudes.

The establishment of attitudes which are conducive to health is one of the objectives of health promotion (see Section 5.3). It is therefore of central importance to consider what attitudes are and how they can be changed. The relationship between attitudes and behaviour, and situational influences on this relationship, are of particular interest. Are attitudes predictive of behaviour? Will a change in an attitude necessarily result in a change in behaviour? And conversely, is attitude change a prerequisite for behavioural change? What factors affect these relationships?

It should be made clear from the outset that attitudes cannot be examined and measured in a direct, standardized manner such as might be employed to measure blood pressure, body mass index, or physical fitness. Rather, we can only infer what attitudes are held through exploration of related traits such as beliefs and behaviour. Moreover, it is often necessary to identify attitudes within a particular context. Attitudes are characteristics of individuals, but they are influenced and determined by many societal and situational (as well as personal) factors. An understanding of the range of factors which influence attitudes, and how these interact, is central to the development and delivery of effective health promotion action.

It is important that these issues are examined, not least because we have to be clear about the consequences which can realistically be expected from programmes which effect a change in attitudes.

7.1 What is an attitude?

A number of definitions of an attitude exist, of which we shall examine two. Roediger *et al.* (1984; p. 587) define an attitude as 'a relatively stable tendency to respond consistently to particular people, objects, or situations'. This definition raises several points.

First, attitudes are *'relatively stable'*; they are not fixed, and therefore, they change and can be changed. Secondly, the phrase *'respond consistently'* implies that a person's behavioural response in a situation provides an indication of their attitude towards it. By observing someone's behaviour it should be possible to deduce their attitudes. However, the qualifier that it is a *'tendency to respond consistently'* indicates that it is possible to behave inconsistently with one's attitudes. A person's behaviour does not necessarily represent those attitudes in a straightforward manner.

There are three reasons why this may be so. The first is that a person's attitude may on some occasions not lead to the corresponding behaviour because a strong desire may lead to action inconsistent with the attitude. For example, a person may have a favourable attitude towards losing weight, but be overcome by a strong desire to eat rich food. Of course, if such desires consistently dominate the person's behaviour we may come to doubt the existence of the favourable attitude towards losing weight. (An occasional lapse is consistent with the existence of the attitude, although lapses make inferences from behaviour to attitudes uncertain.)

The second reason for the uncertainty of inference from behaviour to attitude is that people have many attitudes, and these may on occasion conflict. For example, a favourable attitude to losing weight may be held at the same time as a favourable attitude to courtesy, or to a specific host, and the result may be that a rich meal is accepted, inconsistent with the favourable attitude to diet but consistent with the favourable attitude to courtesy.

There is a third reason why a person's attitude, or intent to behave in a particular way, may not result in the corresponding behaviour being shown. The attitude-related behaviour may not ensue if it conflicts with social, cultural, or group norms; if it is discordant with the behaviour expected in a particular situation or by the dominant social or cultural ethos of the occasion.

These exceptions do not contradict the phrase 'a tendency

to respond consistently' but they alert us to situations where behaviour may be inconsistent with attitudes.

The definition states, thirdly, that an attitude is a 'relatively stable tendency to respond consistently *to particular people, objects, or situations*'. In other words, an attitude must be *towards* something. This raises the question, 'Can an attitude be held towards anything?'. The answer is 'yes', although it seems trivial to talk about holding attitudes towards some things. An important point is that it is possible to hold an attitude towards another attitude. For example, an elderly person may have an attitude of fear or anxiety towards falling or being left alone, but at the same time have an attitude of contempt towards the first attitude. Those dealing with elderly people will be familiar with the problems such conflicts of attitudes may bring with them. Conflicts of attitudes of this kind can, however, be helpful, as we shall see later, in bringing about attitude change, for where a favourable attitude towards health exists it provides something on which health education can get a grip in order to weaken potentially unhealthy attitudes.

The definition given by Roediger *et al.* may be compared with the fuller definition of Ribeaux and Poppleton (1978): 'an attitude is a learned predisposition to think, feel and act in a particular way towards a given object or class of objects'. If we now examine that definition, several issues are of interest.

First, an attitude is a '*learned predisposition*'. Now, it is true that learning is sometimes a conscious process involving understanding, but sometimes we 'learn' without noticing that we are doing so. Similarly, an attitude may be changed as a result of consciously acquired knowledge and understanding, but this is not always the case. For example, a person's attitude towards painkillers may be changed by an advertisement for a new product which 'relieves pain faster'. He or she does not need to learn *why* the new product relieves pain faster in order to hold a favourable attitude towards, and be more likely to buy, the new product. It seems, then, that attitudes are not necessarily *consciously* 'learned predispositions'. Rather, they might sometimes be more accurately said to be 'acquired'.

Attitudes are acquired on the basis of some experience or evidence, either direct or indirect. For example, a favourable attitude towards the new painkiller might be acquired through direct experience that it does 'relieve pain faster', or through indirect evidence of being told that it does so. What is clear is that attitudes are not fixed at birth, but rather are acquired in some way at some stage in life. In this sense, they are clearly distinct from instincts.

Ribeaux and Poppleton's definition also states that an attitude is a *'predisposition to think, feel and act in a particular way'*. There are three aspects, then, to an attitude—the cognitive, or belief aspect; the affective, or feeling aspect; and the conative, or behavioural aspect. So, as with the Roediger *et al.* definition, an attitude is seen to be related to behaviour. In addition, however, cognitive and affective aspects are said to be present. We can regard the cognitive aspect as an active, conscious belief, the affective aspect as a non-rational, gut-reaction feeling; and the conative aspect as observed behaviour.

The two definitions examined here represent distinct viewpoints. That of Roediger *et al.* may be regarded as unidimensional. It focuses on only one component of an attitude, namely 'the tendency to respond'. No indication is given of different classes or types of response. Ribeaux and Poppleton's definition, on the other hand, is a three-component model of attitudes. Indeed, it goes beyond defining an attitude, and gives an indication of attitude structure. The three components appear separate but are not completely unrelated.

There are contradictory conclusions from the research that has been carried out to test which of these two models provides a more accurate description of attitudes (Chaiken and Stangor 1987). The unidimensional model is that most frequently adopted, for simplicity, in attempts to measure attitudes. For other purposes within the field of health promotion, the three-component component model seems to be the more useful. We shall now examine the three components in more detail, with respect to health-related attitudes.

The *cognitive component* concerns the individual's belief about an object or attitude. This belief may not be a true or accurate representation of the facts—it may be biased or incomplete. But it represents the individual's own direct or indirect intellectual evaluation of the object, based on facts collected or acquired.

As we have said, however, beliefs are not always based on the weight of objective evidence; they can also be based on inaccurate personal estimations. From the point of view of health promotion this latter aspect is the more important and the more problematic (Tones 1981). While it has been found to be a relatively straightforward task to change people's *general* beliefs about health-related behaviour, their beliefs about *their own* susceptibility to disease or the effectiveness of interventions are less easily changed. For example, most people have been convinced by frequent presentations of the evidence that there are impressive correlations between smoking and lung cancer, but some people continue to believe that, in their particular case, smoking will not cause lung cancer on the grounds that, say, a grandfather or neighbour smoked all his life and lived until he was ninety.

Personal estimations of evidence (which are expressions of the cognitive component of an attitude) are also influenced by, and themselves influence, the *affective component* of an attitude—feelings, likes and dislikes, and emotions. The affective component is also important for health promotion. For example, a child may correctly believe that the eating of sweets or sugary foods can damage teeth. Nevertheless, the child may like sweets, experience enjoyment when eating them, and therefore eat them. Indeed, there are a great many situations in which our emotions and our likes and dislikes, override what we know or believe to be the sensible (or healthy) course of action.

A person's feelings are also influenced by his or her values. A great deal more will be said about values in Chapter 9, so it is sufficient here to state that our values are about how things *ought* to be, and serve as the standards by which we assess the way things are. The affective component of an attitude, then, is concerned not with an intellectual evaluation of the situation but with feelings about it, and such feelings can be influenced by the value system which we hold.

The *conative component* is the behavioural component of an attitude. The term 'behaviour' takes in a wide range of phenomena, verbal and non-verbal, including consciously effected actions and even physiological reactions. These events also take place within a range of environmental situations which will themselves influence behaviour. There is difficulty, then, in assuming that what a person says or does is an accurate reflection of his or her attitude. A distinction has been drawn, for example, between attitudes and opinions (e.g. Wheldall 1975). An opinion is a publicly stated expression of an attitude, but the true attitude held may only be expressed in situations where there is trust and privacy. Thus, opinion polls are exactly that, and cannot be taken as an accurate and valid indication of people's true attitudes.

The foregoing analysis is helpful in highlighting the three main components of attitudes, each of which may be taken as an indicator of the attitude that is held. It is important to stress, however, that all three components are not necessarily present in a concordant or consistent manner. There are a great many situations where people's beliefs and feelings are positive (for example, towards the benefits of exercise), but they behave in a contradictory way (have an inactive lifestyle). The possession of an attitude does not necessitate that the person thinks, feels, and acts in a particular way. All three aspects are not necessarily present.

In addition to having the three components described above, attitudes have several *dimensions*. We have already implied, firstly, that attitudes have *direction*, that they are positive, negative, or neutral. We can now develop this characterization by adding further dimensions, beginning with extremeness and strength. *Extremeness* refers to the extent of direction, to how positive or negative the attitude is. *Strength* can be regarded as an indication of the stability of an attitude, of its resistance to change. It is a product of extremeness together with the length of time for which the attitude has been held, and like extremeness it is also affected by the individual's own personality, the attitudes of the reference groups to which the subject belongs, and the degree of integration of this attitude with his or her other attitudes. A fourth dimension of attitude, the degree to which it is related to and integrated with other attitudes, is known as the *isolation* of the attitude. The less isolated an attitude, the more resistant it is to change.

A fifth relevant dimension is the *cognitive content*. People may hold the same attitude but for different reasons. For example, a positive attitude towards a new painkiller will have a shallow cognitive depth (and be relatively unstable) if it has arisen solely as a result of seeing the television advert for it. It will have greater cognitive depth (and be relatively stable) if it has arisen from a knowledge of biochemical innovation from which the painkiller has resulted. Finally, attitudes have a sixth dimension of *differentiation* or sophistication. This is a measurement of how clear or structured the attitude is.

Each of these six dimensions—direction, extremeness, strength, isolation, cognition, and differentiation—affects the stability (or resistance to change) of an attitude; and the complexity of their interrelationship provides an indication of the problems to be faced when trying to effect change in attitudes.

A different characterization of the dimensions of attitudes and behaviour was presented by Ajzen and Fishbein (1977). They identified four specific elements:

- the *action* element (i.e. *what* behaviour is to be performed)
- the *target* element (i.e. *at what target* the behaviour is to be directed)
- the *context* element (i.e. *in what context* the behaviour is to be performed)
- the *time* element (i.e. *when* the behaviour is to be performed).

They argued that observations of a lack of correlation between attitudes and behaviour are sometimes due to the fact that measurements made of the two often do not correspond in their degree of specificity in relation to the four identified elements. This issue is explored further in Section 7.3.

7.2 Attitudes and health promotion

Given the complex nature of attitudes—their many dimensions and relationships to other personal traits including beliefs, feelings, values, and behaviours—it is clear that attention to attitudes will strengthen health promotion action, whether or not attitudinal change is a specific objective of that action.

Particularly important in this respect is the recent work of Kelly (e.g. Kelly 1992; Kelly and Sullivan 1992), based on the stress-coping paradigm of Lazarus (1976, 1984). Kelly argues that the perspective of the patient (or, for health promotion programmes outside the health service setting, the public) must be taken into account, otherwise programmes may yield unintended consequences which can reduce their effectiveness. Attention needs to be paid to the imagery and meaning of health promotion initiatives. The danger is to assume that the meaning taken by the recipient will be the same as that ascribed by the health promotion specialist.

The health promotion initiative can be regarded as a potentially stressful event for its recipient—not because of the content of the initiative or event *per se*, but rather because of the way people perceive or define it. Thus, to understand the process, we should examine not merely the health promotion intervention itself, but how people appraise it. We need to know whether the intervention creates a threat, or whether it is regarded as benign, positive, or irrelevant. If it is regarded as a threat, we must equip people with the skills to deal with that threat.

In other words, an intervention which creates fear or threat can be a positive or effective intervention—as long as a means of dealing with the threat is provided at the same time. An appreciation of the recipient's beliefs and attitudes (as well as other aspects of their situation) is integral to understanding how they will appraise the health promotion intervention, and cope with the stimulus if it is regarded as stressful.

An understanding of *the processes of threat and coping* should be applied not only to the primary target group (or 'recipients' of an initiative) but also to secondary audiences. This is particularly important when we are concerned with attitudes towards sensitive issues such as sexual behaviour. Many sexual health promotion campaigns for young people have collapsed because they have failed to take account of the attitudes of other—often powerful and influential—sections of society. The important point is not that initiatives must always suit everyone—'you can't please all the people all of the time', but rather that if an intervention is likely to be perceived as threatening by a section of society, then that section should be presented with ways of coping with it. Sometimes the provision of factual information will be adequate in this regard.

It follows that for effective health promotion it is necessary to consider not only the attitudes of the lay public, but also those of key players, including policy-makers. In Section 3.1 we have highlighted the important role that policy-makers have to play in health promotion, the necessity to view them as a key target group for health education, and the extent to which they can act either to facilitate or to inhibit health promotion action at local, national, and international levels. Moreover, the variation in attitudes of key players (and the organizations that they represent) in alliances for health is the basis of many of the challenges that confront us in inter-sectoral working. For healthy alliances to be productive, stakeholders need to be prepared to examine their own attitudes and to move beyond the viewpoint or stance characteristically taken by the organization that they represent. Only when a common set of attitudes towards health promotion is established will the commitment be there for agencies to work truly collaboratively in alliances and bring their expertise and resources to bear towards the achievement of a common aim.

In discussions of attitudes, there has been a tendency to focus on how someone feels about characteristics of others, or a new service, or some aspect of society. However, increasing recognition is now being given to the importance of the attitudes that people hold *towards themselves*. These include self-esteem, self-perception, health locus of control, and self-confidence. Several of these attitudes have been found to have a strong positive association with health-enhancing behaviour. Recognition of these associations forms the basis of much of the lifeskills focus of modern health education (see Section 3.3.3).

One attitude to self that has been viewed as worthy of attention, particularly in relation to the uptake of preventive services and behaviours, is that of *perceived susceptibility* or vulnerability. The concept of perceived vulnerability is an integral component of the Health Belief Model (Becker 1974). This model postulated that perceptions of being susceptible to some condition, the perceived seriousness of the condition, and perceptions of the relative costs and benefits of behaviours that prevent or treat the condition are all related to the likelihood that an individual will engage in some specific preventive behaviour. Perceived susceptibility has been regarded as the most important of the three variables (Gochman and Saucier 1982).

Models such as the Health Belief Model and the more recent Health Action Model (Tones 1979) provide valuable representations of the factors and process which influence health-related behaviour, and their interactions. Attitudes are integral to both these models—although positioned rather differently in each.

An appreciation of the role and position of attitudes in influencing health action is valuable not only when planning and implementing health promotion programmes, but also with respect to their monitoring and evaluation. Within the framework of a behavioural science model, attitudes can be measured prior to intervention and changes to attitudes predicted and monitored in relation to changes in other components of the model. A *systems approach* such as this is required if we are to move beyond a simple single focus for health promotion programmes. Attitudinal change may be of interest in itself, but it is likely to be of much more interest if it can be seen to relate to changes in behaviour (whether of the individual him/herself or of others) or in health status (whether self-perceived or objectively measured).

In order to be able to monitor attitudinal change, and appraise its impact on other factors, we need to be able to measure attitudes in a valid and reliable manner. It is to this issue that we shall now turn our attention.

7.3 Identifying and measuring attitudes

As we have seen, attitudes have many facets and manifestations, and are affected by a range of personal and situational factors. Their measurement is, therefore, not a straightforward process.

Given that the cognitive, conative, and affective aspects of an attitude need not coincide, and indeed do not all need to be present, if measurement focuses on only one manifestation it may yield a distorted or misleading picture of the situation. Given the several dimensions of an attitude, how can we be sure of what it is we are measuring? Further difficulties include the facts that there is no universal agreement on the nature of some attitudes ('self-perception', for example); and that fluctuating or less strongly held attitudes cannot be reliably identified by information gathered on only one occasion.

When we measure attitudes, we must rely on *inference*. It is impossible to measure attitudes directly. Henerson, Morris, and Fitz-Gibbon (1990) identify four approaches for gathering information about attitudes. These are as follows:

1. **self-report measures**, whereby members of a group report directly about their own attitudes;
2. **reports of others**, whereby others report about the attitudes of members of the group of interest;
3. **sociometric procedures**, whereby members of a group report about their attitudes to one another;
4. **records** that provide information with attitudinal implications.

Whatever approach is used, the identification of attitudes depends on making inferences from what people say and/or from how they behave.

The first method—*asking directly* what attitude is held—is problematical in that the response received will reflect personal and situational factors, as well as the subject's true feelings. For example, when asked to state their attitude towards something, people often offer the response which they think is the 'correct' one, or which they think the interviewer 'wants to hear'. It is possible, however, to formulate questions in such a way that this problem is minimized.

Self-report measures form the most direct type of measurement and are ideally used in conjunction with other methods, as a means of validation. They are nevertheless usually recognized as the measurement of choice as long as the subject has the self-awareness to recognize personal beliefs and feelings, has the ability to express them, and has no reason to lie.

Asking others about the attitudes of the individuals or groups of interest is a useful approach when we are concerned with attitudes which are strongly expressed through behaviour. Observations of others are generally regarded as more credible than retrospective self-reports—as long as the reporter is in a position of objectivity, and has had a complete, not partial, view of the behaviour of interest.

When measuring attitudes, either through self-report measures or through reports of others, the most common tools involve *attitude rating scales*. These yield a score which indicates both the direction and intensity of a person's attitude. Some scales can also yield sub-scale scores. For example, within a rating scale measuring attitudes towards cigarette smoking, subscale scores might relate to attitudes towards smoking at work, attitudes towards smoking in social settings, and so on.

The most commonly used attitude rating scales are agreement scales, based on the approach developed by Likert (1932). In a *Likert scale*, a series of attitude statements (including extreme statements clearly favourable and unfavourable) is presented, and respondents are asked to indicate their strength of agreement or disagreement with each statement. A graded scale is provided, which is balanced around a neutral point and has the same number of positive and negative symbols. Usually a five-point scale is used, ranging from 'strongly agree' to 'strongly disagree'. An attitude score is computed by totalling the respondent's answers to different items.

The two other principal methods used in attitude scale construction were developed by Thurstone (1928) and Osgood *et al.* (1957). The *Thurstone method* has an interval structure (whereby it is assumed that the difference between two consecutive points is equal to the difference between any two others) and is often represented graphically, as a ladder or thermometer for example. *Osgood's semantic differential technique* is based on a series of bipolar ratings (defined by adjectives and their antonyms) which describe a person's attitude to the object in question.

An alternative to asking questions about the attitude held is to *observe people's behaviour*. Observation of behaviour is not without its difficulties, however, since it assumes that behaviour is a true reflection of the attitudes held by a person. We have already illustrated that this is not necessarily the case—the behavioural component of an attitude is not always present and, even when it is, it is not necessarily concordant with the other components of the attitude.

In some situations, however, behaviour is reasonably regarded as a true reflection of a person's attitude—and a more useful indicator than a self-reported attitude measurement. For example, while patients may be reluctant to express their dissatisfaction with new procedures introduced by their GP in their Health Centre, if they uncharacteristically fail to reattend the surgery, or if they change their doctor (and there are no other particular reasons why they should do this), we might reasonably assume that they hold a negative attitude towards the new procedures.

In other situations it matters less what people say they would do; it is what they actually *do* do that affects policies. Thus, even if opinion polls indicate that a large proportion of the community wants to use an existing sports facility, if attendance figures are too low to indicate a demand, then the facility may no longer receive financial backing.

It may, of course, not be possible to determine attitudes by observing behaviour. We may want to *predict* how people will behave under a new condition (such as the provision of a totally non-smoking bar) or we may want to examine attitudes to some totally hypothetical situation (a completely private health care system, for example). In cases such as these the first method—direct inquiry—is the only possible one.

Whatever approach is taken to identifying and measuring attitudes, it needs to be sufficiently complex not only to identify which attitudes are held but also to determine their strength and stability. Measures also need to be valid and reliable (see Chapter 5). If attitudinal change is a major objective of an intervention then the evaluator cannot rely simply on one measure of attitudes, nor on measurement at only one point in time.

7.4 Attitude change

The most useful theories for explaining attitude change are *cognitive consistency theories* based on Heider's theory of consistency (Heider 1944). The argument is that people strive to have their own 'cognitions' (beliefs, attitudes, and perceptions) organized in a tension-free manner. Tension arises when cognitions are contradictory, resulting in the person being motivated to bring them into a tension-free state. We shall examine two theories of cognitive consistency: balance theory and cognitive dissonance theory.

According to Heider's *balance theory* (1958), tension alone is not sufficient to generate attitude change—the individual must become aware of the imbalance. When imbalance is discovered there are three possible types of outcome:

1. the direction of one or more of the cognitions can be changed;
2. one or more of the elements can be redefined;
3. the individual can cease to think about the matter and thus restore cognitive consistency.

Imagine, for example, the position of the schoolboy who discovers that his role models smoke cigarettes but who himself believes that this is an unhealthy, unattractive habit. He is in a state of tension because people for whom he has great admiration and respect (and towards whom he has strong positive attitudes) are displaying a pattern of behaviour which he regards as dangerous and unpleasant (towards which he has strong negative attitudes). To reduce this state of tension he may, in the first instance, decide that cigarette smoking is not unhealthy and unpleasant after all, and thus change the direction of his attitude towards smoking. In the second instance he might redefine the behaviour of his role models by deciding that what they are doing is not in fact smoking cigarettes in a dangerous and unattractive way—perhaps they are not inhaling the smoke, or are just going through a 'phase': they are not really 'smokers'. His third option is to ignore the inconsistency. Balance theory does not predict which of these outcomes will occur.

Cognitive dissonance theory was proposed by Festinger (1957) and differs from balance theory in that it includes actions. People's attitudes are taken to determine their behaviour. When attitudes conflict, or conflict with behaviour, cognitive dissonance results in a change of attitudes or behaviour such that they come back into harmony. Cognitive dissonance theory helps us to predict what will happen when people are forced to do or say something contrary to their private belief. For illustration we can refer to an experiment by Festinger and Carlsmith (1959), as follows.

Two groups carried out boring, pointless tasks. Group A were paid $1 and told to inform the next subject that the tasks had been fun and interesting. Group B were paid $20 to do the same thing. When asked afterwards for their opinion of the interest of the task, it was rated higher by the $1 group than by the $20 group. According to cognitive dissonance theory, Group B could justify lying to their successors because they were adequately rewarded in doing so. For Group A, on the other hand, the sum of money involved was so small that it did not justify lying. They could not explain their lying behaviour by reference to the external factor of a reward. Consequently, they experienced dissonance as a result of lying about the boring tasks. The dissonance was resolved by redefining the tasks as interesting.

Cognitive dissonance theory also enables us to make predictions about the way in which people expose themselves to information. It predicts that people seek information in such a way as to maintain cognitive consonance, or avoid cognitive dissonance. They are motivated to expose themselves to attitude-consonant information (that which is concordant with their existing attitudes) and to avoid attitude-dissonant information. This *selective exposure hypothesis* has been supported by research findings (e.g. Frey 1986). This research also identified the conditions under which people act contrary to the selective exposure hypothesis, and expose themselves to dissonant information. They will do so either when their cognitions are relatively weak, and it seems better to change them to be consonant with the information; or when their cognitive system is strong, and they can argue against new information and accommodate it in balance with existing attitudes. These research findings have important implications for health promotion strategies for attitude change.

It follows from our understanding of the importance of cognitive consistency that the creation of dissonance or imbalance is a potentially effective mechanism by which to achieve attitudinal (and/or behaviour) change. Attitudes can be changed in two main ways: by the provision of information or experience inconsistent with current beliefs, or by making people behave in a manner which is inconsistent with their beliefs.

Provision of information is the foundation of health education action and is, undoubtedly, the most commonly adopted health promotion methodology. Information is provided to individuals or groups through a variety of media including written materials (leaflets, booklets, magazines, newspapers, etc.); the spoken word through radio, audio tapes, or personal contact; or in a visual manner by film or television. The mere repeated exposure of an individual to a stimulus has been shown to be sufficient to enhance his or her attitude towards it (Zajonc 1968). Nevertheless, people are bombarded daily with a mass of information and only a small proportion of it ever 'sticks'. The aim, then, is to present information in a way that will be attractive and have immediate impact, and causes it to be accepted and retained.

There are several factors involved in the provision of information for attitude change. These can be summed up by the phrase, 'who says what to whom and in what way'. In this phrase, 'who' is the communicator, 'what' is the communication or message, 'whom' is the audience, and the 'way' is the medium of communication. For each of these components, the key features which have been associated with a successful outcome can be summarized as follows.

7.4.1 The communicator

— A message is more likely to be accepted if it is delivered by someone who has similarities with the audience, and who is honest and sincere about the message he or she is putting across.
— Messages are often more effective if they are overheard rather than directed towards the listener (Walster and Festinger 1962). People become suspicious if they think that the communicator is trying to persuade them of something.
— The greater the prestige possessed by the communicator, the greater the change in attitudes he or she is likely to produce. People are not foolish enough to believe information just because it is told to them. They need to have some basis for judging its credibility.
— The processes of peer pressure and peer support are recognized as playing important roles in influencing attitudes and behaviour. The

use of group members, peer educators, or opinion leaders within a community as a source of information can thus be an effective strategy.

7.4.2 The communication

— The information must be useful and relevant to the audience. Information is much more likely to be attended to and retained if it has relevance for the person at that moment.
— Positive information is preferred. People attend more to good news than bad, especially when they are forming an opinion or when their commitment to an opinion is low. If fear-inducing approaches are used, then the communication also has to involve means for enabling the audience to cope with that message (see Section 7.2).
— The message should be put in a simple way. Information often fails to get across because it is too complicated.
— Novel or alternative methods can increase the impact of a communication. The audience is more likely to change attitudes on the basis of new information. However, arguments or methods of presentation which are too extreme for an audience should be avoided. Anything that differs too much from current beliefs is likely to be rejected.

7.4.3 The audience

— In general terms, the more important the issue is to the audience, the more they will be affected by the quality of the argument presented rather than by 'secondary' factors such as aspects of the communicator, the environment, and so on.
— Audiences who feel that they have made up their minds freely on a given subject are more resistant to changing their opinions than are those who feel that they had little choice in their decisions.
— Subjects who are persuasible under one set of conditions tend also to be so under others (Hovland and Janis 1959). It is not clear what personality factors are responsible for this tendency, although self-esteem, gender, and intelligence are all thought to play a role.
— Other 'receiver factors' which will affect the effectiveness of attempts to change attitudes include the amount of motivation receivers have to attend to the message; their memory and comprehension of the message; the consequences of the attitude change for them in terms of reward or punishment; and their perception of the amount of pressure acting on them towards conformity both to (sub-)cultural norms and to their own personality type. Whilst most of these factors are outside

the communicator's control, some of them may be alterable in his or her favour.

7.4.4 The communication medium

— The written word provides a medium for presenting a case in its entirety, without interruption. Its big advantages are its relative permanence and visibility, anonymity for the audience, and its usefulness in a range of settings and situations. It depends, however, on a degree of literacy and comprehension, and provides no scope for discussion, clarification or questioning.

— Audiovisual modalities are most effective if they incorporate some of the ingredients for success already identified: presentation by a credible, prestigious presenter with similarities to the audience, giving positive information honestly and in a simple and relevant form. Use of audiovisual methods may, however, be restricted by availability of resources, and also by the physical aspects of the setting. Audiovisual communications can also become dated more rapidly than do written materials.

— Use of the mass media has clear advantages when it comes to providing information to vast numbers of people. Moreover, they reach those groups in society with fewer material and cultural resources (Medrich 1979), and who are thus key target groups for health promotion messages. Use of mass media can be very expensive, and may be limited in terms of targeting particular sections of society. However, the mass media are extremely powerful communication mechanisms.

— Evaluations of the effectiveness of mass media campaigns have shown that while mass communication may be very useful by itself, its effectiveness is greatly enhanced if it is combined with other methods of communication (e.g. Maccoby and Farquhar 1975). Where the ideal balance lies between community-based, face-to-face interventions and high-profile, faceless mass media initiatives is open for debate. According to Maccoby and Alexander (1980) the best strategy 'blends a minimal but focused amount of face-to-face instruction with an extensive media campaign that is strong enough to create the desired outcomes, in part, by itself (p. 369). Others, for example advocates of a Healthy Cities type of approach, would tend to see mass media campaigns as having a very limited role, largely in support of the community development and interagency work being carried out on the ground.

The alternative approach to providing information as a means of achieving attitude change, is to encourage people to *behave* in a manner which is inconsistent with their current beliefs (*counter-attitudinal behaviour*). There are situations in which it is clearly impossible, or unethical, to change behaviour for the purpose of changing attitudes. For example, one cannot make people directly experience a nuclear winter in order to change their attitudes towards nuclear weaponry; nor is it ethical to prescribe addictive drugs such as heroin or morphine to people in order to create an understanding and change attitudes towards the plight of drug addicts. However, in many cases it is possible to adapt people's behaviour, or to create a situation whereby people have to behave in a particular way.

Health promotion approaches to adapting behaviour include methodologies such as role-play, experiential learning and drama. Clearly these are labour-intensive methods and are limited to small groups. Nevertheless, they have been found to be effective in changing people's attitudes (including attitudes to self) and perceptions. Moreover, the change has been relatively long-term in nature. These methods are, therefore, regarded as promising as means for changing attitudes. Good quality interactive health education recognizes the value, where possible, of going beyond the provision of information to the implementation of approaches for the adaptation of behaviour.

An alternative to behaviour adaptation is that of creating environments or situations which facilitate or even necessitate the adoption of behaviours conducive to health. Such approaches are integral to the health protection sphere of health promotion (see p. 52).

At its extreme, health protection involves *legislation* to make people behave in a particular way. If they do not behave according to the law, they will be punished. This is a powerful argument when trying to make people behave contrary to their own desires—and also provides a mechanism (or excuse) for the 'macho' to modify his behaviour.

Legislation has been found to be an effective health promotion measure in certain circumstances. Most notable in recent years has been the seat-belt legislation in the UK. Legislation was crucial to the achievement of universal seat-belt use—and thus to the reduction of serious and fatal road traffic accidents—but it is widely believed that the success of the legislation owes much to the pioneering 'Clunk-Click' campaign that was fronted by Jimmy Savile. This campaign to educate the public preceded the legislation and ensured that the public was properly prepared.

Pinet (1987, p. 88) has emphasized the importance of public education prior to legislation: 'A law, even the soundest one, that does not have public support, cannot be implemented.'

Legislation is, of course, only one health protection approach for achieving behaviour change, and as an approach is limited by a great many procedural and political factors, as well as influences of powerful lobbies, economic factors, and ethical issues (see Chapter 10). More common approaches involve the *introduction of policies or practices* at a local level, to create environments whereby particular behaviours are inhibited or forbidden, and thus other behaviours are facilitated. Workplace smoking policies are one example.

Local experience in Glasgow, for instance in relation to the Health Board's own smoke-free policy, has been that despite the existence of strong negative attitudes towards the proposed policy held by a minority of staff, subsequent to the introduction of the policy these negative attitudes became much less strong and were held by a smaller minority. The policy's introduction produced no-smoking behaviour in line with the policy's requirements, and thereafter a change of staff attitudes in line with the patterns of behaviour being expressed.

This approach, of creating environments whereby health-enhancing behaviours are facilitated, and thereby yielding attitudinal change concordant with health promotion, is increasingly being recognized as invaluable. Even though exposure to the health-enhancing environment may be limited, concordant behavioural and attitudinal change in that environment are very likely to yield health-promoting changes in other situations.

7.5 Conclusions

1. Attitudes are central to our understanding of people's behaviour. Attitudes are affected by beliefs and values and may be reflected in feelings and behaviour.
2. Attitudes are relatively stable entities, but are not fixed. They change and can be changed.
3. Attitudes are acquired through personal experiences, the main influences being the immediate primary groups such as family and friends, although secondary influences such as the school, and peer or reference groups are also extremely important to the formation of attitudes.
4. Attitudes have several functions. They enable us to filter and order

our experiences, and can also justify or support our behaviour, as in the case of attitudes of disbelief held by smokers. Moreover, we can attract attention by expressing certain attitudes rather than others. If these attitudes are approved by others, this results in reinforcement and consequently these attitudes will increase in strength.

5. People's attitudes will influence how they perceive and deal with health promotion interventions, particularly if the intervention is potentially threatening. Attention therefore needs to be paid to the imagery and meaning ascribed to health promotion initiatives by their recipients.

6. Identification of attitudes held can be carried out either by direct questioning or by behaviour observation. Each method has disadvantages, but care with methodology can increase the reliability of results.

7. Psychological theories of attitude change bring out the complex nature of these concepts. Attitudes can be changed by a challenge to the knowledge or value base, or by altering people's behaviour. Both of these approaches have been employed in health promotion initiatives.

8. Key principles for increasing the effectiveness of approaches for changing attitudes have been identified in this chapter. Workers in the field are likely to raise their chances of success by noting the types of recommendations made.

8 Objections to health promotion

In the preceding chapters we have offered an analysis of the nature of health, suggested a model of health promotion, and outlined and illustrated various methods of health promotion and their attendant difficulties. It must be admitted, however, that health promotion has its critics. In the end the only satisfactory way to meet these criticisms is to provide a value-base for health promotion, and this task will be carried out in the next three chapters. Before beginning the task, however, it will be helpful to look explicitly at these objections and provide some preliminary answers. It will be remembered that the model of health promotion (see p. 59) identified three connected and overlapping component activities—health education, prevention, and health protection. The objections to be considered, while they may be aimed in general terms at health promotion, usually have one or other of the components as their main target, and in replying we shall therefore identify the particular aspect of health promotion at which the objection is being directed.

8.1 Standard objections

In general terms, the objections to health promotion fall into seven main groups, which overlap. First, there is the claim that health promoters adopt a sneering attitude to conventional medicine, or the 'biomedical model'. This we shall call the objection of 'moral superiority'. Secondly, another kind of comparison with clinical medicine is developed. It is said that whereas in clinical medicine patients on the whole *request* interventions, and the clinical imperative correspondingly requires that 'something must be done', even if it is only to give advice or reassurance, in health promotion there may be no requests. How then, or to what extent,

can intervention be justified? Are health promoters simply interfering busybodies? Screening programmes are sometimes included
in this kind of attack. We shall call this the objection of 'gratuitous
intervention'. Thirdly, it is alleged that health promotion (unlike
medical treatment) is ideological. It is not only guilty of gratuitous
intervention but it is also pursuing a particular set of values which
not everyone shares, and some people might reject. In their
pursuit of this ideological agenda health promoters run the risk
of being labelled 'health fascists'. Fourthly, there is the claim
that health promotion employs such a wide conception of health
that health engulfs every good human state—well-being, fitness,
self-esteem, empowerment, fulfilment . . . Correspondingly, every
good human activity—going for a swim, listening to a symphony,
taking a holiday, getting the council to repair the leaking roof—
can count as health promotion. This is the objection of 'health
imperialism'. Fifthly, it has been argued that health promotion
encourages obsession with one's own health states. This is the
objection of 'self-absorption'. Sixthly, health promotion has been
said to adopt the methods of its opponents, bypass our autonomy
and sell health like a commodity. This is the objection of 'health
commercialism'. Finally, there is the objection, applying especially
to health promotion work in schools, that even health *education* is
really 'health indoctrination'.

8.2 Moral superiority

Medicine is often criticized for having too narrow a view of health
and its determinants. What is called the 'biomedical' model of
health presents health in negative terms as the absence of disease,
injury, or disability (p. 10) and sees health interventions primarily
in terms of 'treatments' for existing conditions. Mencken (1923) put
the points in this way: 'The aim of medicine is surely not to make
men virtuous; it is to safeguard and rescue them from their vices'.
On the other hand it is sometimes suggested that the aim of health
promotion just is to make us virtuous. In terms of this contrast
we can compare medical interventions and health promotion as
follows.

First, medicine characteristically bypasses our rational minds
and treats us as causal mechanisms. In other words, characteristic
medical treatments are biochemical or surgical, whereas health

promotion, among other things, characteristically attempts to enable us to understand our bodies and their environment. Secondly, medicine typically (but again by no means exclusively) stresses the curative or palliative, while health promotion stresses the preventive and embraces positive health. Going along with the second distinction we might say, thirdly, that medicine stresses the health needs of individuals, whereas health promotion tends to have a broader societal perspective. Fourthly, and perhaps most fundamentally, medicine tends to be reductivist in its assumptions—this follows from the scientific study of disease processes on which it is based—whereas health promotion tends to be holistic in its assumptions.

But can it be construed from these distinctions, if they contain at least some truth, that health promotion is viewed by its proponents as being in some way ethically superior to medicine? This by no means follows: there is a place for both approaches. What does follow is that health promotion gives rise to an acute set of ethical problems because it is interfering with lifestyle. It therefore requires considerable ethical justification. This we shall provide in the next three chapters.

8.3 Gratuitous intervention

The second common objection to health promotion involves a different kind of contrast with clinical medicine. The single most important factor in the clinical encounter is what we might term the clinical imperative, which states that in the doctor–patient relationship 'something must be done'. 'Something must be done' because the patient has *requested* help. This 'something' may be nothing more than patients telling their story and the doctor responding verbally in an appropriate and helpful fashion, or it may involve the whole gamut of modern technology; nevertheless *something* must be done in response to the patient's needs and demands.

But the clinical imperative, it might be said, does not apply to health promotion. For any specific intervention (legislation for clean water, a programme of immunization, restrictions on smoking in public places, or whatever), the necessary precondition of implementation is that it will improve the health of the public—and this improvement must be *objectively* demonstrable. In this context, as distinct from the clinical context, no patient is requesting intervention: experts are deciding that intervention is necessary and the onus is therefore on them to establish the need for intervention. According to this approach, effectiveness must be established by scientific means, such that all rational and competent judges can agree on the facts. The most common technique for establishing effectiveness of this kind is through the discipline of epidemiology, a difficult and demanding discipline, and one in which clear and certain conclusions may not always be obtainable. Other ways of establishing the effectiveness of health promotion can also be found in the literature (p. 77).

In contrast, there has been little requirement for clinical medicine to be objectively effective. Although some parts of clinical medicine are of established scientific value (those parts, for example, proven by double-blind, randomized controlled trials, or rendered at least probable by clinical success), this does not extend to the whole of medical practice, nor do the results of even the most rigorous group study ever apply exactly to the infinite individual diversity of clinical experience. But whatever the current state of clinical science might be with respect to a given problem, 'something must be done' to help the patient.

Consequently we can outline the difference between the ethics of clinical medicine and those governing health promotion. In the one case the ethics flow from the imperatives of a face-to-face encounter with a suffering human being; in the other they regulate the optional application of scientifically established interventions designed to improve the health of populations who may not have demanded the changes (Kelly and Charlton 1992).

Against this background, the advice given and other action taken in health promotion must be based on sound evidence—it must be demonstrable, for instance, that exercise or a low fat diet are health determinants, or that preventive measures such as screening are effective. In these areas some precision is possible, but health promotion can reasonably be criticized ethically if it extends beyond its expertise in those areas (Skrabanek 1990). Let us look at screening in particular.

Screening can be defined in various ways, but a simple definition is provided by Stone and Stewart (1994): 'Screening is a preventive activity which seeks to identify an unsuspected disease or pre-disease condition for which an effective intervention is available'. Screening is currently a fashionable medical activity. The demand for it is being encouraged by the UK Government

and by certain patients' organizations. Politically it seems desirable because there is a belief that prevention saves money, and
successive governments have therefore set up various screening
programmes. For example, a national screening programme for
the prevention of cervical cancer was set up in 1964, and for breast
cancer a national screening programme was established in 1988 for
women aged 50–64 years. The establishment of such programmes
has been enthusiastically supported by various women's groups.
Indeed, such is the current demand for screening that Shickle and
Chadwick (1994), in a discussion of the ethics of screening, ask
whether 'screeningitis' is an incurable disease. If it were such no
doubt there would be a demand for a screening programme!

It is possible to screen for many conditions, but screening
programmes must satisfy ethical criteria. First, they must satisfy the criteria for any sort of medical intervention. Secondly,
since screening initiatives tend to be profession-driven rather
than individual-driven, there is an additional responsibility for
the professional to justify the intervention which may not have
been requested. Thirdly, the summons to attend for screening
will generally be directed to symptomless individuals. But some
screening procedures carry health risks, and all of them are likely
to be accompanied by discomfort, anxiety, and inconvenience.
Fourthly, any screening programme carries with it the risk of the
false positive or the false negative. For these reasons—there may
be others—screening requires as much ethical justification as other
medical interventions. Moreover, since screening programmes are
expensive they require evaluation.

It is interesting to note that, although the main growth of writing
in the area of medical ethics began in the 1970s, the criteria for
screening were drawn up by Wilson and Jungner and adopted by
WHO in 1968. These criteria are a sensible mixture of the medical,
the ethical, the economic, and the democratic. They are listed
below as principles 1–10. In 1992 the Ad Hoc Group on Screening
Research added a further four principles (which had already been
proposed by Professor Haggard of the MRC Hearing Research
Unit at Nottingham). These are added below as principles 11–14.

1. The condition sought should be an important health problem.
2. There should be an accepted treatment for patients with recognized
   disease.
3. Facilities for diagnosis and treatment should be available.
4. There should be a recognizable latent or early symptomatic stage.

5. There should be a suitable test or examination.
6. The test should be acceptable to the population.
7. The natural history of the condition, including development from latent to declared disease, should be adequately understood.
8. There should be an agreed policy on whom to treat as patients.
9. The cost of case-finding (including diagnosis and treatment of patients diagnosed) should be economically balanced in relation to possible expenditure on medical care as a whole.
10. Case-finding should be a continuing process and not a 'once and for all' project.
11. The incidental harm done by screening, and by the information (correct or otherwise) that it gives, should be small in relation to the total benefits from the screening–assessment–treatment system.
12. There should be agreed guidelines on whom to divulge the provisional and final results to, and on when and how this is best done; there should be transitional counselling support where necessary.
13. All screening arrangements should be reviewed from time to time in the light of changes in demography, culture, health services, technologies, and the epidemiology of the target conditions.
14. Since 'cases' are not homogeneous, the balance of costs, benefits and risks from screening, assessments, and treatments has to be worked out on a stratified (demographic or case-type) basis.

8.4 Health fascism

A nastier variant of the 'gratuitous intervention' objection to health promotion is the 'health fascism' objection. It is that health promotion is attempting to impose a certain lifestyle on us whether we want it or not.

Now, while this way of putting the objection is exaggerated and over-dramatic, it has some elements of truth. The health promotion movement is value-driven in a way in which medicine is not. It is committed to the view that there are better and worse ways of living one's life, and that there are better and worse ways of organizing society and distributing its goods and services. In other words, health promotion has moral and political commitments. For example, in our discussion of well-being (pp. 18–20), we distinguished between subjective well-being—the well-being of a passing mood—and true well-being which is rooted in empowerment. Health promotion is committed to encouraging the kinds of actions which will bring about true well-being. But this is not to say that there is only one correct way of leading one's life. The health promotion position is the modest one that some sorts of behaviour and some social and political arrangements are much more likely than others to bring about true well-being. A modest position of this sort is hardly health fascism.

8.5 Health imperialism

Those making the charge of health imperialism might argue that what in health promotion terms is 'positive health' is really just a name for a range of states which are as easily or better seen in other ways. For example, 'well-being' is just another name for happiness, and there are no professional skills which can assist us to attain happiness. Again, the idea of 'fitness' might be said to be a technical one, relative to specific ends, such as playing professional football but not one with an important bearing on health. The charge of health imperialism can be directed also at mental health. Mental illness may satisfy some of the criteria for illness (although even that has been disputed) but positive mental health might be said by critics to be a concept which attempts to annex the territory of the well-adjusted to that of the healthy. For example, mental illnesses, such as depressions or obsessions, are incapacitating in a manner similar to physical illness, but to stress positive mental health might be seen as simply making a value-judgement in favour of the conventional or the well-balanced as opposed to the eccentric.

The reply to the charge of health imperialism can be expressed in terms which are partly logical or philosophical and partly practical. There is a philosophical view going back to Plato which can be conveyed by the slogan 'Everything is what it is and not another thing'. According to this view it must either be true or false that well-being or fitness are components of the concept of health. But concepts can be much more flexible than this. Indeed, it may only be concepts in exact sciences which are rigid and mutually exclusive. Many concepts overlap, or are 'open-textured'. For example, the concept of an opera will overlap with that of a musical. Again, one and the same phenomenon can be seen in different ways for different purposes. For example, a morning assembly at school can be seen as an occasion for making announcements or as an expression of corporate identity. In like manner, for certain purposes, or in certain contexts, it is helpful to include well-being or fitness in the concept of health, whereas in other contexts it might seem inappropriate to do so. In other words, there is no correct answer to the question 'Is well-being really part of the concept of health?' For example, two people who have acknowledged their love for each other may experience states of well-being, but it would be a comic distortion to construe this purely in terms of health.

Turning now to the activities which critics might claim represent the imperialism of health promotion we find that the same kind of conceptual flexibility is helpful. For example, suppose that a local authority builds a leisure complex with swimming pool, gymnasium, cinema, and so on. Is this a health promotional enterprise or not? Again, there is no one answer to this question. From one point of view it could be seen as contributing to prevention or health protection, fitness or well-being, but from another it might seem too solemn to see it in these terms; rather it is a centre where people can have fun.

Through alliances for health, facilities of this sort can be designed and provided in such a way that they make wide-ranging contributions to health promotion (see p. 73). However, they can be viewed as having value in their own right, without recourse to the contexts of health or health promotion. If such arguments are borne in mind by protagonists of health promotion, the charge of health imperialism can be avoided.

8.6 Self-absorption

We must concede that an undue concern with physical health is a characteristic to be found in some present-day societies, perhaps especially on the west coast of the United States. But to see health as a positive good is not necessarily to commit oneself to self-absorption. It is certainly the view of the WHO that positive health is 'seen as a resource for everyday life, not the objective of living'. The point is that positive health is a value, not the supreme value. It makes perfectly good sense to weigh health against other values, and sometimes it will be reasonable to give precedence to health and sometimes not. For example, someone with a stressful lifestyle might give up a job—perhaps at some personal economic cost or even to the detriment of service to others—on the grounds that his or her health was suffering. Equally, someone might reasonably sacrifice health for another value, such as dedication to a life of scholarship or service to others. To say that health is a value and makes a claim is by no means to say it is the supreme value or requires self-absorption.

8.7 Health commercialism

The sixth sort of objection to health promotion is that it attempts to bypass autonomy and to sell health like a commodity. In this it might be said to resemble the advertisements for unhealthful products which it is opposing (Williams 1984).

In reply to this argument we might question the premise that all true education respects autonomy. It might be maintained that autonomy is not something which everyone in fact possesses. People can be victims of all sorts of social processes and be lacking in power. It is quite unrealistic to regard all recipients of health education as autonomous. Education of any kind, whether concerned with health or not, must take into account the fact that people, young or old, must be 'empowered', and education is an important part of the process of empowerment. It must aim at creating or enhancing autonomy, but should not presuppose it. This issue is ethically important and must be examined in more detail. Is health education really 'education' or is it rather 'training', 'instruction', or even 'indoctrination'?

The criteria for calling an activity 'educational' have been worked out in much detail in the many writings of R. S. Peters (1973), and it is illuminating to look at health education in the light of the distinctions he drew between 'training' or 'instruction' on the one hand and 'education' on the other. It should be said that Peters developed the distinctions in slightly different ways in different works, and what is offered here therefore is more of a paraphrase of his distinctions than an expression of any one way in which he drew them.

The first and most important criterion is that something worth-while or valuable for its own sake must be passed on in any activity which is properly to be called education. It is obvious that Fagin's class in picking pockets in Dickens's *Oliver Twist*, while it may have been training, could not be regarded as education, because it was actually harmful to others. There are also neutral activities which may count as 'training' but are not 'education' in terms of Peters's distinction. A student, for example, can be trained to give an intravenous injection, but this is not education although the technique when learned can be used to help a patient. In terms of this distinction teaching on health may or may not count as 'education'. To the extent that we concentrate on the practical uses of health education, we are thinking of it as training for a further end—such as cutting down expenditure on health care, improving the efficiency of industry, reducing the number of days off work, and so on. But to the extent that we stress the intrinsic value of the human biology and behavioural sciences involved in health education, and the intrinsic value of health itself as a component in a good or flourishing human life, we are seeing it as a part of education.

The second criterion which any activity must satisfy if it is to be educational is that it must have wide cognitive perspectives. Thus, activities such as science, history, literature, and so on are central to education, not only because they are valuable in themselves but also because they may deepen and widen one's understanding of other matters. Imagine, for example, a historian of the French Revolution who was surprised when he was told that a study of this period led people to think of such matters as social justice, and said that he was just interested in 'the facts'. It might be more appropriate to say of such a person that he had been 'trained' as a historian than that he had been educated as one. In terms of this criterion we can again look at health education in different ways, depending on how it is taught and at what level. If it is taught as a set of 'tips' for healthy living then it is instruction or training, but it can be taught at a higher level with wide cognitive perspectives.

The third criterion which any educational activity must satisfy, besides being valuable in itself and related to other activities thought valuable, is that those engaged in it must come to care about what they are doing. Suppose that students have completed courses in biology or literature (activities which are valuable in themselves and have wide cognitive perspectives) but thereafter show no interest in these subjects. We might say that they have been highly trained or instructed but, if they do not care about what they have studied, they are not educated. In terms of this criterion health education can count as part of education. Indeed, one of the main points of health education is to encourage people to care about their health, to view health as a value in its own right regardless of its usefulness.

Fourthly, education implies that a person's whole outlook has been transformed—it involves 'wholeness—whereas training suggests a competence of more limited scope. In terms of this criterion health education can count as education. Indeed, in terms of this criterion it does better than many subjects traditionally regarded as part of education. Health is such a central aspect of human existence that if people can be brought to value their own health and that of their community in the context of the commercial and environmental threats to it, their outlook will really have been transformed. Education, as distinct from training, has to do with opening out, with 'educing', with releasing and liberating. This is one realistic possibility for health education, and one which makes it ethically worthwhile.

Fifthly, it follows from the previous point that the educator must employ different methods from the trainer or instructor. It is consistent with training or instruction, for example, to use methods based on fear, threats, indoctrination, or hidden persuasion. By contrast, the educator must always use person-respecting methods; education must encourage critical thought and must be a two-way process.

However, as we have already stressed, we must not exaggerate the extent to which human beings are autonomous, rational, and critical thinkers. In view of the political and commercial power of the anti-health forces in society, health must be presented in as attractive a way as possible or health education will fail. If health educators confine themselves strictly to the rational, critical approach to education, then it is preferable to depict health education as the element within a larger health promotion movement concerned with health advocacy, legislative change, fiscal reform, and the mobilization of community interests as well as education narrowly conceived.

The tension between the ethical requirement to be person-respecting in methods and the practical necessity to be effective is addressed from an interesting point of view in the literature of self-help groups. The growth of self-care groups concerned with a range of maladies and involving both the sufferers and their relatives has been a notable development during the last decade. These movements avoid the charge of paternalism commonly still made against every branch of health care, including health education.

Apart from ethical considerations, self-care movements seem to be effective within their limits, although they may benefit from a professional health educator to advise and facilitate. Advising and facilitating do indeed constitute an important role for health education.

Let us now sum up this discussion as to whether health education is really 'education'. The argument has been that health education can be genuinely educative. In terms of its content and its method it can pass on something worthwhile or valuable for its own sake, it can have a wide cognitive perspective, it can encourage its students to care about health and so transform their outlook, and it can use person-respecting methods, although it is important that these methods should be appropriate for young children or for those at risk from anti-health movements.

8.8 Health indoctrination

The charge that the health promotion movement is involved in indoctrination is not convincing if we think of it as targeting adults, or so we have argued in the previous section. But what about children? There can be objections even to health education as it may be presented in schools (Downie and Fyfe 1990). It is sometimes argued that, despite what we have claimed for education, health education involves ethical and political indoctrination and in this respect is therefore not person-respecting. Now, it is true that some health education approaches take an overtly political stance. Examples include discussions of governments' roles in relation to the promotion of unhealthful products through advertising, and because of the taxation benefits. Publications such as *The smoke ring* (Taylor 1985) identify the roles of specific named MPs in endorsing unhealthy products. Does discussion of the political dimensions of health involve indoctrination?

Different models and conceptions of health have resulted in a range of alternative views about the remit of health education. It is, therefore, important for health educators to clarify the parameters of their concerns if they are to be effective in practice. Now, it is widely known that the influences on health are multifactorial, and include environmental and political factors.

Indeed it has been stated that the *fundamental* determinants of health and health care are political. If we accept the importance of political influences on health, we should then accept that discussion of these influences should play a role in health education.

It does not follow, however, that the inclusion of a political aspect turns health education into indoctrination. Person-respecting methods must still be used, and the distinction between 'politics' and 'party politics' remembered. Education about the political aspects of health must involve the learners in critical assessment of the facts, not merely unquestioning acceptance of one particular viewpoint. Young people are certainly able to understand and assimilate arguments concerning the role of advertising, the political sway of large multinational companies, and so on. Discussions about these issues should certainly be a component of health education in schools, and cannot reasonably be thought to offend against the ethical requirements of educational method. Obviously such discussions are suitable only for more advanced pupils.

Contrary to the fear of the inclusion of political dimensions within health education is the argument that health education in schools at present does not take a *sufficiently* political stance. Cribb (1986) describes the forces which press towards a conservative curriculum. These include the examination system, the lobby for traditional academic subjects, the argument that education should be relevant to the marketplace, and the stress placed on the primacy of basic expository skills. He argues, however, that schools are not independent from politics, that teachers should examine and become self-conscious about the values which they are transmitting to their pupils, that 'teaching for political literacy is not only different from the transmission of ideologies, it is a positive safeguard against it'.

We agree with this view. Young people are being exposed to many influences which are not free from bias and distortion, and a role of school health education should be to raise their critical awareness of these issues. It should not merely sweep them under the carpet. Children being educated to value health must consider all aspects and the range of known determinants of health. Health education should change their way of seeing the world.

8.9 Conclusions

1. A number of characteristic objections are often levelled at health promotion, which we have labelled: moral superiority, gratuitous intervention, health fascism, health imperialism, self-absorption, health commercialism, and health indoctrination.
2. These objections, which apply in complex ways to the expertise, the messages, and the methods of health promotion, can be answered, although they serve as warnings to over-enthusiasm for health promotion.
3. A full understanding of health promotion requires an explanation of its value base.

9 Values

In Chapter 7 we discussed the nature of attitudes and the various ways in which they may be changed. This immediately raises the question of the direction in which they ought to be changed. In other words, it raises the question of values. The question of values in the context of health promotion is complex. We shall try to analyse the nature of values and valuing, the nature of the values which are necessary if an individual person and a society are going to flourish, and the bearing which the activities of health promotion have on these values. These questions, which are often glossed over in the literature, are of the first importance for a proper understanding and justification of health promotion, as we stressed in our account of health in Chapter 2.

9.1 Terminology

One of the difficulties in the literature of health education and health promotion is that terminology varies. We have already encountered this in the discussions in Part 1. Terminology for discussing values is particularly varied. This is partly because health promotion is an eclectic discipline which draws from a range of social sciences, from health care sciences of all kinds, from traditional moral philosophy, and from lay perceptions. It is also partly because health promotion is attempting to forge its own concepts to express its own distinctive insights.

Sometimes this confusion is a simple matter of new words for old ideas. For example, we shall speak here mainly of 'self-development' where we have previously stressed the importance of 'acquiring lifeskills'; and in this chapter we shall stick to the traditional emphasis on the importance of developing 'autonomy' whereas we previously spoke of the importance of 'empowerment'. We therefore ask our readers to consider whether the terminology which comes easily from their own professional approach can be

translated into this terminology without loss. In a new and rapidly
developing discipline it is important to be tolerant of a variety of
approaches and terminology.

Confusion can also extend beyond terminology to the values
which lie behind it. Once again, the fact that several currents
of thought and concern flow into health promotion is important. For example, the medical values of public health, and the
educational values of traditional health education, mingle with
newer values of consumerism and 'getting the message across'.
We shall try to clarify the value stance of health promotion
in this chapter and the next, and we shall try to clarify the
political stance of health promotion in Chapter 11. In attempting to do this we shall no doubt express our own moral and
political position, but we shall try to show that the moral and
political values of health promotion derive from its intrinsic *professional* concerns rather than from any extraneous non-professional
reasons.

The word 'ethics' is more familiar in the wider literature of health
care than 'values', so the question arises as to why we are making
the term 'values' central. The term 'ethics', despite its frequent
use, has no clear or consistent use in the literature of health care
(Downie and Calman 1994) but it is sometimes used to refer to
the first-order problems which are encountered in the practice of
health care. We shall use the terms 'value' and 'value-judgement'
here rather than either 'ethics' and 'ethical judgement' or 'morals'
and 'moral judgement'. There are three reasons for preferring
this usage.

First, it brings out the continuity between the value dilemmas
encountered in ordinary life and those dealt with in the professional
practice of health promotion. The point here is that the activity of
health promotion is one which can be approached from numerous
professional standpoints, such as medicine, dentistry, nursing,
education, and social work. What these various professionals
have in common, and can bring to health promotion, is their
sense of judgement as ordinary human beings informed and
sensitized by their professional backgrounds. Certainly, there
is a growing knowledge-base to health promotion, but it is vital
that health promotion should not develop as a new kind of
esoteric expertise divorced from the values and ideas implicit
in lay perceptions of health and a good life. If we think in this
way of health promotion, as an activity of 'enabling', 'articulating',

'crystallizing' or 'refining and mobilizing' the values implicit in lay perceptions, or of 'empowering' individuals, then it is preferable to use terms which emphasize the continuity with ordinary situations. We are therefore proposing to speak of 'values' rather than 'ethics'.

A second reason for preferring the term 'values' to 'ethics' is that it emphasizes the essentially contestable nature of the practice of health promotion. The term 'ethics', especially in the context of medical ethics, is apt to suggest the unchangeable principles of hallowed tradition; a body of rules written on tablets of stone by the Greeks, and nowadays developed by committees of 'experts'. But this spirit is quite alien to the practice of health promotion. Public involvement and debate are essential in all areas of health promotion, and a 'top-down' approach is undesirable. To use the term 'values' rather than 'ethics' is to suggest that differences of approach and emphasis are desirable.

Thirdly, the term 'values' brings out much more clearly than the term 'ethics' the breadth of the problems involved. For example, in Chapter 10 we shall raise as a problem of values the priority which should be given to individual freedom when that is an obstacle to community health. Clearly, such a problem is wider than anything conceived within the framework of professional ethics. Again, we consider, in various contexts, concepts such as self-development or social justice. Discussion of such concepts involves information which derives from a range of social sciences, but it also involves value-judgements, although perhaps not 'ethical judgements' in the narrow sense.

In summary, we can say that while specialist health promoters may in time develop a code of ethics to regulate their professional practices, it is preferable to think of their activities as being essentially concerned with values and value-judgements. This is because the term 'values' brings out the continuity between the work of health promoters and our own ordinary judgements of good and bad forms of individual and social life; it brings out the essentially contestable nature of the activities of health promoters and therefore the importance of public participation in the debate about values; and it brings out the breadth of the value-base of health promotion. We must also be alert to the wide variety of terms, professional and lay, which are used to express values.

9.2 What are values?

To answer this question we may consider first what kinds of thing are naturally spoken of as a person's values (Downie and Telfer 1980). We say, for example, 'My values (or 'my values in life') are integrity, kindness, beauty'. Does this just mean: 'These are the things I value?' No, because I may value highly my car or my hiking boots, but it would be odd to say that these things were among my values, except as a joke.

This is not a moral point about the triviality of having such things as one's values. Rather it is a conceptual point about a person's values. In the case of a car or hiking boots, we can always ask why someone sets such a high value on such things, and get an answer in terms of more general considerations. For example, a woman may say she values her car because it gives her freedom or excitement, and she may value her hiking boots because they are comfortable. But where something is to be regarded as among a person's values, no further reason can be given why these things are valued. If kindness is among a person's values then it is valued for its own sake, and other things (e.g. a thoughtful letter) can be valued as exemplifying the fundamental value.

Can we then say that a person's values are simply those things which are valued *for their own sake*? This is not very informative without further discussion of what it is to value something. Now, a great deal has been written on this, but a fairly rough-and-ready characterization will do for our present purposes. We might try the approach that valuing is to do with preference and choice; to value something more highly than something else is to choose to have it or get it in preference to the other thing, to choose to hold on to it in preference to the other thing, and so on.

Described in this way valuing is essentially comparative—we value by comparing and then choosing—whereas simply having certain values does not seem to be so. But we can accommodate the apparent non-comparativeness of what are said to be a person's values in terms of the comparative notion by saying that a person's values are those things which for their own sakes are preferred to everything else. Thus, if health is among a person's values, he or she will sacrifice other things in order to achieve health, unless another value is also at stake or the person is weak-willed.

But this account of valuing fails to distinguish between two distinct ways in which something might be valued for its own sake. The distinction is best explained by means of an example. Suppose an independent, elderly man takes a lot of pains to live on his own, sacrificing all sorts of possibilities in order to maintain his independence, apparently with no further end in view—we would then say that independence is one of his values. Now there are two possibilities. On the one hand, he may say that he happens to like independence but is happy to let others stay with relatives or enter institutions. On the other hand, he may disapprove of those who depend on others, and try to bring up his children to set the same store by independence as he does himself. Again, a man who values thrift and enterprise for their own sakes may either simply like to be thrifty and enterprising, as a matter of temperament; or he may approve of thrift and enterprise in himself and others, be ashamed of himself if he is extravagant or unenterprising, and so on. We can call the first kind of values 'liking values' (though liking will be too mild a word to convey the strength of some valuings of this kind), and the second kind 'moral values'. When people speak of values they more often mean moral values, and if we use the word 'values' without qualification we shall be referring to moral values.

Both liking values and moral values affect people's conduct; they lead them to act, inspire their conduct, and have a bearing on their attitudes, as we saw in Chapter 7. But moral values, as distinct from liking values, have an interpersonal quality. People with a particular moral value will judge others as well as themselves in terms of it. That is the source of the attitudes of approval and disapproval which are characteristic expressions of moral values. We shall later consider (Section 10.3) whether 'health' is a liking value or a moral value.

We are now in a position to raise the question of the relationship between values and attitudes. The answer is that values—both liking and moral values—are subsets of attitudes. Attitudes, we said, have cognitive, affective, and conative components. The same is true of values, which are expressed in *behaviour*, and through *preferences* based on *beliefs* about objects, persons, or situations, and are accompanied by *feelings* of approval or disapproval. For example, some individuals may judge that conduct likely to risk the spread of AIDS is wrong. This means that they choose one mode of behaviour rather than another because they entertain certain beliefs about the spread of AIDS and the harm it may cause themselves or others, that they disapprove of others who act in high-risk ways, and feel guilty if they themselves do so. In other words, having a value is the very same as having a certain sort of attitude.

Values, then, are preferences which both express attitudes and affect attitudes. The relationship may be conveyed as follows:

9.3 Necessary social values

It is often maintained that values differ enormously in different societies and in different parts of the same society. This view is sometimes expressed by saying that values are 'relative' to a society, or, even more drastically, that they are 'subjective' and personal to the people holding them. We wish to argue that this view is exaggerated. Whereas some values have changed historically, and there are differences over many values in different areas of contemporary society, there are also other values which are widely shared, and indeed *must* be widely shared for the continuance of society. There are other values again which are necessary for individual human flourishing. We shall consider the latter in Section 9.4, but let us begin by considering the sense in which some values must be adopted or accepted, or must develop, in any continuing society. These we regard as consensus values, and they are the very same as those which constitute the collective dimension of the social well-being of the WHO definition discussed in Chapter 2.

One approach to the idea of consensus values is to describe in general terms the human predicament for which the existence of consensus values is the partial solution. The description of human nature and its predicament we shall give will consist of a few obvious truths about human nature. Such a description brings out the close links between the kind of nature we have and the kind of values we have. To say this is not to say that values can be deduced from the facts of human nature, but rather that we accept the kind of values we do because we are the kind of people we are, that any plausible account of values must have close links with an account of what people and their environment are like. It will emerge that because people and their environment have certain characteristics, obvious to us all, they must observe certain rules or constraints on their behaviour—or not survive. In other words, we are assuming that whatever may be the full analysis of consensus values, they at least give rise to principles which help us to live together more harmoniously and co-operatively than we otherwise would without such principles. To say this is not to deny that values may have a spiritual dimension, but it is to assert that they have a social function, and that we have an interest in accepting certain principles of behaviour.

As a first example of how an obvious fact about human beings gives rise to principles of behaviour let us note that human beings have bodies and minds which are vulnerable both to attack and disease, and are easily damaged by either. This obvious physical fact, which we examined in detail in Chapter 2, is the basis of the values of physical integrity and health and the disvalues expressed in concepts like 'assault' or 'illness'. These values give rise to rules and customs, found in any society, which restrict the use of physical violence in social life and minimize the risk of disease. A concept like 'assault' logically could not exist unless the human body were liable to physical damage. And, in more general terms, principles such as 'One ought not to harm', or 'One ought to help people in distress' clearly reflect the facts that people are liable to injury and are vulnerable physically to deliberate attacks, accidental mishaps, and diseases.

Less obviously, but just as importantly for our purposes, human beings are vulnerable to psychological pressures of all sorts. Sometimes these may be inflicted by social forces, such as economic constraints. This obvious fact lies behind many of the campaigns for social justice, for the constant threat or reality of poverty damages human beings. The human psyche is vulnerable also to damage from gossip or patronizing behaviour, or to self-inflicted feelings of guilt or inadequacy. As we shall see, such obvious facts about human beings lie behind many of our basic values as to how people should be treated in society. For example, the health promoter's stress on building up self-esteem reflects such facts. Indeed, health promotion in general, as we stressed in Chapters 2–4, is concerned with facilitating true well-being in adverse physical and social circumstances.

Secondly, human needs and wants can more adequately be satisfied co-operatively by division of labour, than by each fending for himself. These facts are reflected in the complexities of social and economic organization, with its value of justice, which we shall discuss in Chapter 11. Other concepts important for health promotion, such as 'neighbourliness', 'citizenship', and 'self-help', can also be seen to reflect basic human needs and wants.

Thirdly, human beings are approximately equal in most respects. Some people are stronger or cleverer or more attractive than others, but on the whole these natural gifts tend to balance out, giving us all an interest in accepting principles which work for the benefit of all.

Fourthly, human rationality is limited, and rules are therefore helpful to guide us on the likely consequence of action. J. S. Mill (1861) said that rules are like signposts which guide us when we are not sure where to go, or they distil the wisdom of mankind on the consequences of action.

Fifthly, human sympathy exists—by nature we have the germs of benevolence or compassion within us—but our benevolence is limited and easily swamped by the stronger natural endowment of self-assertion in all its forms. We recognize this in each other and therefore have an interest in belonging to a system of morality, the principles of which correct our bias towards self-interest.

Finally, the resources of the environment are scarce and require work for their production and distribution through service industries. Scarcity gives us an interest in property and in the many rules of justice for the legitimate ownership and fair transfer of property and other goods and services, including health care.

These six facts put together explain why we have an *interest* in accepting a system of social values or why a consensus is desirable. For it seems to follow from such obvious natural facts that, on the whole, we will all do better for ourselves by belonging to a system of organization which reflects the consensus values. Of course, not everyone accepts those values, and changing circumstances modify them, but a majority accept them. This is especially so when the values are enshrined and safeguarded by a system of law and legal sanctions.

The most basic of these principles which derive from what we have called 'consensus values' are the following:

1. One ought not to harm other people physically or psychologically (non-maleficence).
2. One ought to give positive help to people wherever necessary (benevolence or beneficence, and compassion).
3. One ought to treat people fairly or equally before the law, in the ownership and transfer of goods and services, rewarding labour, and in general in determining social conditions (justice).
4. One ought to produce the best possible consequences (or the greatest happiness) for the majority (utility).

These values can all be seen to be acceptable to human beings, granted the limitations already mentioned of human nature and the human situation. And of course these four consensus values will give rise to many detailed rules of helping others—property rules, rules of fair dealing, and many more. In the next two chapters we shall consider how these values and principles of social life are or ought to be the guiding principles or 'ethics' of health promotion in various social, personal, and educational contexts. In other words, if these are the values which constitute societal well-being, they must also be the values which health promotion is attempting to nurture.

9.4 Necessary individual or personal values

Let us now turn from social values to individual or personal values. Again, just as we maintained that there are some social values which must be widely shared if societies are going to operate on a harmonious and co-operative basis, so we maintain that there are some individual and personal values which are necessary for a good, in the sense of flourishing, individual human life. Once again, the fruitful question is not 'What values do individuals in fact have?' but rather, 'What are the values which are components of a flourishing human life?'

One important and widely shared personal value can be called the ability to be self-determining, the ability to be able to choose for oneself or, more extensively, to be able to formulate and carry out one's own plans or policies. The importance we attach to these abilities is reflected in our approval of traits of character such as 'being able to stand on one's own feet', 'knowing what one wants', 'having aims in one's life', or 'being able to make up one's own mind'. The connection between developing such traits of character and being a person is reflected in theories of education which stress the importance of cultivating such dispositions in children. Conversely, to impair a person's abilities to formulate and carry out aims and policies of his or her own devising is to that extent to injure him or her as a person. For example, if a person has been injured physically or mentally there is often a tendency for friends to offer too much help, for it is often easier to do something for people than to wait patiently while they try to do it for themselves; and this ease and convenience can assume the guise of kindness. But it may be a subtle way of eroding someone's nature as a person. The development of personality can also be blocked in grander ways by political arrangements which restrict the images people can form of themselves, or by consumer societies which impose certain images of people. Self-determination, then, is a personal value essential to the growth and development of the human personality and therefore to true well-being (Downie and Telfer 1980).

A second value which is important for the integrity and flourishing of human personality we can call the ability to be self-governing. Philosophers such as Kant have attached great importance to this value, and have certainly exaggerated the extent to which it can actually be realized in most people's lifestyle, granted the many economic and psychological pressures on them in their everyday lives. Nevertheless, it is correct to say that the ability to be detached, to stand back from one's own self-interest, to take account of the needs of others as well as of one's own—in short, mould one's conduct in terms of values applying to all equally—is one mark of the mature personality.

A third value to which individuals attach a great deal of importance, and which is necessary for a mature personality, we can call a sense of responsibility. Human beings assume that they are responsible for their actions, unless in some way they are compelled to act as they do, or they do not understand what they are doing. Approaches to human beings which ignore or deny this factor, such as some medical, psychiatric, or social work interventions, can be experienced as patronizing and an affront to human dignity.

A fourth personal value to which people attach importance we can identify in general terms as self-development or self-realization. Most people feel that there are some activities—physical, mental, social—which they are or could be good at. This awareness goes along with a desire to develop the capacity or express it. Sometimes this may take the form of what we have earlier called a 'liking value'. For instance, some people have a capacity for a sport, and they wish to develop this or express it by actually playing. At other times the awareness of this capacity may take the stronger form of what we have called a moral value; some people feel that it is morally incumbent on them to develop their gifts for their own sake and not because the gifts may be useful to others. An example of this is the person of mature years who leaves a job in order to begin a course of full-time study which will not necessarily lead to a better job but may lead to self-development and thereby improved self-esteem. That this preference is a moral value, and not just a liking value, is indicated by the fact that sometimes a person will feel justified in sacrificing the interests of family or friends for it. In other words, a desire for self-development can at times outweigh a social value. We shall later consider the relationship between health and self-development.

Some philosophers deny that there can be a self-regarding side to morality, such as we are identifying via the concept of self-development. They see morality as having an essentially social function, concerned only with regulating one's conduct *vis-à-vis* other members of society. Such a view has developed out of one strand in J. S. Mill's thinking. Mill (1859) in his essay *On liberty* seemed to be arguing that moral issues arise only to the extent that one's conduct harms other people; in so far as one's conduct affects only oneself it does not raise a moral issue. Yet in the same essay Mill has a chapter on 'self-development', in which he does not seem to regard it as a matter of moral indifference what kind of person one is. As he puts it (in his Chapter 3): 'It really is of importance not only what men do, but also what manner of men they are that do it.' And this view, that there are moral duties to cultivate in oneself certain characteristic human excellences, goes back to Plato and Aristotle, and is taken up in a slightly different form by the Judaeo-Christian tradition. In other words, self-development has been regarded as a morally important attitude from the earliest.

We have already noted in this chapter that there can be alternative terms for the same concept. The literature on health education and health promotion recognizes the importance of what we have called 'self-development' by its stress on the importance of acquiring 'lifeskills'. In particular, lifeskills involve learning how to make decisions, to take control of one's own life, rather than be at the mercy of circumstances (see pp. 31, 37). Other writers (e.g. Antonovsky 1984) stress the importance of acquiring a 'sense of coherence' in one's life. These and no doubt others are overlapping terms for what we are identifying as 'self-development'.

It might be objected that we have said little in this chapter about self-esteem, a concept much stressed in the health promotion literature. But self-esteem is not a value in its own right because it cannot be chosen. What can be chosen is self-development, or, in more typical health promotion language, the development of lifeskills. Now if a person chooses to develop lifeskills then self-esteem will result. In other words, self-esteem is a by-product of lifeskills. It is a sign that self-development is going well, rather than an aim.

9.5 Autonomy

These four values—self-determination, self-government, sense of responsibility, and self-development—are clearly linked. For example, self-development will often be achieved by exercising self-determination. In other words, we develop the self by achieving certain purposes or acquiring lifeskills. Again, people often feel responsible for their failure to develop their gifts and blame themselves. In view of the overlapping and connected nature of these personal values it is helpful to regard them all as being different aspects of a single concept—autonomy. The concept of autonomy is often used in the literature of medical, nursing, and social work ethics, but less commonly analysed. We are suggesting that it encapsulates the four important personal values of self-determination, self-government, sense of responsibility, and self-development.

It is important to make three further points about the autonomous person, as we understand the value of autonomy. The first is that we are not excluding as unimportant human emotions and desires. It will be remembered that we have maintained that values are a subset of attitudes. They have therefore a cognitive, an affective, and a conative component. In so far as autonomy is the unifying value of individual personality it too will have all three aspects, and thus will have an affective aspect.

The second point which must be stressed about the autonomous person is that he or she is a kind of abstraction from a social situation. Human beings do not exist in complete separation from each other. The ingredients of autonomy all carry an essential reference to society. Our self-determination, self-government, sense of responsibility, and self-development are not only emotionally charged but also exist only in a social context and cannot really be understood without that dimension. The autonomous self is a social self.

Politically this means that the autonomous person is a citizen—his or her nature and values cannot be understood outside a political and economic framework. Emotionally it means that the autonomous person does not live in a vacuum; persons exist in emotional relationships with others and these relationships are essential to their identity. As we shall show in the next two chapters, there are messages to be learned from this for health promotion.

The third point, which is made many times in this book, is that autonomy is a *value*, an ideal to be aimed at rather than a characteristic which everyone possesses. People are frequently prevented—by social and economic forces, by pressures from commercial interests or peer groups—from developing their capacity for autonomy. Health promotion is one movement which contributes to the development of autonomy. That is why health promoters often express their professional aims in terms of the concept of empowerment. To empower people is to enable them to develop their autonomy, or to 'be all they can be'. This was a central theme of Chapters 2–4.

9.6 Linking social and personal values

From the point of view of our theory of values there is a parallel between social values—the values necessary for the flourishing of society—and individual values, those necessary for the flourishing of the individual personality. It is common in social and political philosophy to depict social values as laying claims upon us, but to depict individual values as being at best 'liking values'—matters of arbitrary preference. Our view is that individual values impose claims on us also. In the case of social values the constraints which make the values *claims*, rather than just *likings*, are the threats of disharmonious and uncooperative social relationships. Analogously, the constraints which make individual values claims are the threats of disharmony and disintegration within the self. Liberal philosophy characteristically stresses the values of avoiding harm to others, and suggests, more or less explicitly, that the self is a structureless receptacle for indiscriminate satisfaction. We, on the contrary, hold that the self has a structure just as society has, and that a sense of coherence and self-esteem, and therefore of true well-being, come from the awareness that the personal values we have mentioned are being expressed in a way of life.

The parallel between social and individual values establishes a link, but only a weak link, between them. Is there any other way of linking them? Kant sees individual and social values as being two aspects of a single principle, which he expresses as: 'Respect the autonomous nature of human beings whether in your own person or in that of another' (Kant 1782).

It is important to stress that Kant thought of it as an obligation to develop in ourselves the qualities which make us distinctively human beings. Most liberal writers are inclined to state the Kantian slogan as: Respect for persons. The implicit suggestion of the abbreviated formula is that it is only *other* persons which are meant. But we are following Kant in thinking that our own personality lays claims upon us; there is a duty to 'be all we can be'.

These basic values can be indicated and linked as shown in the diagram below.

9.7 Conclusions

1. An examination of values is of importance for health promotion because health promotion is concerned with changing attitudes.

The justification for this project clearly involves pervasive value judgements about desirable lifestyles.

2. Values are either 'liking values' or 'moral values' but in either case they are expressions of attitudes and as such have cognitive, affective, and conative components.

3. There are certain consensus values which societies must adopt if they are to flourish. These are the values of interpersonal relationships. Other values are necessary for individual human flourishing. In both cases the values are the expression of obvious physical or psychological truths about human beings and the constraints on their lives, and in both cases the values are the source of the empowerment which constitutes true societal and individual well-being.

10 Liberalism, autonomy, and health

We have discussed in our previous chapter what it is to value something, and have identified the values which are necessary for individual and social flourishing. In this and the next chapter we shall discuss the methods by which health promotion attempts to further the values of autonomy and social justice which we have identified as being necessary for the flourishing of the individual and society. Here it is helpful to state the five principles which WHO (1984) sees as the basis of health promotion.

1. Health promotion involves the population as a whole in the context of their everyday life, rather than focusing on people at risk for specific diseases.
2. Health promotion is directed towards action on the causes or determinants of health.
3. Health promotion combines diverse, but complementary, methods or approaches, including communication, education, legislation, fiscal measures, organizational change, community development, and spontaneous local activities against health hazards.
4. Health promotion aims particularly at effective and concrete public participation.
5. While health promotion is basically an activity in the health and social fields, and not a medical service, health professionals—particularly in primary health care—have an important role in nurturing and enabling health promotion.

We shall try to show in this and the next chapter how these principles can be used to further the values which are essential components of health. In this chapter we shall concentrate mainly on the way they can be used for the enhancement of individual autonomy, and in Chapter 11 we shall consider ways in which they relate to social justice.

It is clear from our view of the place of values in health promotion that we regard it as strongly normative. But not all of those engaged in health promotion share our view that the activity is value-driven. Before considering the way in which health promotion encourages the growth of certain values we must therefore defend our view that health promotion is not a neutral activity. Let us begin by examining the process known in health promotion as 'value(s)-clarification'. This will also assist in further explaining our position on the value-base of health promotion.

10.1 Values-clarification

The term 'values-clarification' refers to processes by which persons or groups can be assisted in finding out what their values really are. There are various methods which can be used to bring about a clarification of this kind (Ewles and Simnett 1985, 1992). For example, people might be encouraged to write down and rank the activities they enjoy, or they might be asked to state the arguments in favour of something they feel strongly about. Again, role-play or games may be used to encourage groups to become clear on their values. Now, the details of these procedures are very important for practical purposes, but we are more interested in the principles and assumptions behind them.

In the first edition of their book on promoting health, Ewles and Simnett (1985) (p. 132) wrote as follows: 'Traditional teaching operates in the hope that the "right" attitudes and values will be "caught" by learners. In contrast, we suggest that health education requires people to think critically about their values and build up their own value system.' Social work literature in a similar vein suggests that in dealing with clients it is important to be 'non-judgemental' (Downie and Telfer 1980). Now, if the assumption here is that any set of values is as good as any other then it is not an assumption which is consistent with health education or promotion, or indeed any sort of education whatsoever. Certainly, it is important that people should be encouraged to think critically about their values, and although our predecessors in health education did not have such imaginative methods as are nowadays recommended for values-clarification there is no reason to think that the encouragement of critical appraisal has not always been part of health education. What does need to be questioned, however, is the phrase 'build up their own value system' and the correlative idea of the non-judgemental attitude.

We are attempting to bring out in the chapters on values that health education and other aspects of health promotion are activities committed to certain views on the nature of the self and what makes it flourish, and to views of a well-ordered society. No doubt there are a large number of acceptable ways of living one's life, all of which lead to the flourishing of human personality, but not *every* way is acceptable. Similarly, there are no doubt several acceptable forms of social and political organization, but not *every* way is acceptable to those involved in health promotion. If these positions are not shared by health educators and health promoters, then why adopt slogans such as 'Be all you can be', or why deplore the 'health divide'? In other words, health promoters cannot consistently accept the 'sneer' quotes in Ewles and Simnett's phrase '"right" attitudes', for health promoters must believe that there are right attitudes to the individual and to society, or go out of business.

It is a totally different point what methods or procedures should be adopted to change attitudes in individuals or societies. Consider this analogy. A Christian missionary priest is not likely to be very successful if he arrives among a heathen tribe and declares 'All have sinned!' He may be committed to believing this, but he would be well-advised to live and work among the people and learn about their ways of life and their difficulties before he tries to change their attitudes. In a similar way, it might be counter-productive to preach too much about giving up smoking or going to the pub every night; but, all the same, a health promoter is committed to the view that smoking and heavy drinking are objectively bad. Again, there may be some doubt as to whether jogging is a desirable form of exercise in all, or indeed in any, circumstances, but there can be no doubt that taking regular exercise is objectively a good form of activity and should be part of a good life. In the area of political values, there can be room for difference of opinion about the relative importance of values such as liberty and equality—we shall discuss this later—but health promoters are surely committed to the view that a large health divide between rich and poor is wrong. But it is a different question of political tactics how this state of affairs is best changed.

Consider this example, again from Ewles and Simnett (1985). In discussing the inadequacies of traditional health education (p. 32) they state that it has sometimes involved (among other failings):

. . . the imposition of medical values on the client. Frequently, this means the imposition of middle-class values on working-class people, and the ethical justification for this is doubtful. For example, losing weight and lowering blood pressure may be the most important thing to a doctor, but drinking beer in the pub with friends may be far more important to his overweight, middle-aged, unemployed patient. Who is to say which set of values is 'right'—the doctor or his patient? Whose life is it anyway?

Two points can be made here. First, if the client wants to lose weight then he ought to take the doctor's advice and cut down on his beer drinking. Otherwise, why consult the doctor at all? Secondly, the health promoter is presumably committed to believing that health is at least one important value, and so is also committed to believing that the client should try to take the doctor's advice. It is a totally different question how the health promoter should go about persuading someone to do this. That question is one of method, on which Ewles and Simnett have many excellent points to make. But if every set of values is as good as every other, then health promoters might as well pack up and go home. It is surely the belief that there are better and worse ways of living one's life that makes the whole practice of health education, promotion, social work, nursing, and medicine worthwhile.

To sum up what we consider to be the underlying principles of values-clarification, we are maintaining three principles: that it is important to encourage people to clarify their own values; that the methods used in doing this should be flexible and imaginative; that health promoters are committed by their profession to believing that there are right and wrong attitudes to life and its values.

10.2 Assumptions of liberalism

In our previous chapter we identified the values which are necessary for the flourishing of individuals and societies. But health promotion takes place in a specific cultural context with assumptions specific to the context about how life should be lived. The framework of values to be found in Britain and the rest of Western Europe, North America, Australasia, and other areas influenced by these can be defined economically, politically, and morally. Economically, this outlook is expressed in some form of free market economy; politically it is expressed in some form of representative democracy; and morally it is expressed in some form of what is called the 'harm principle'—that individuals have a right to act as they want unless they are harming others. (This is often what is meant by 'freedom'.) Taken together these strands can conveniently be labelled 'liberalism' or 'liberal democracy', and they constitute one, but only one, historical embodiment of the values we have identified as necessary for individual and social flourishing.

One important current of thought leading to the modification of some of these assumptions of the liberal outlook is health promotion. In this and the next chapter we shall be discussing the impact of health promotion on liberal ideas. What are the assumptions of the liberal outlook, at least as it applies to health? We shall list the assumptions and then go on to criticize or at least to modify them in the light of the values of health promotion. The liberal position on the pursuit of health assumes the following:

1. A view of health as an instrumental or enabling value, and as not making a claim as a positive value in its own right.
2. The view that people have a right to pursue their own health but no duty to do so unless their ill-health is harming others, this view being thought to be an expression of autonomy, or the 'harm principle'.
3. The connected view that the government has no duty to safeguard or enhance health other than through the prevention of harm.
4. A negative view of health legislation, as restricting autonomy in the interests of health.
5. A negative view of autonomy, that you have it to the extent that you are not prevented from doing what you want to do.
6. An atomistic view of society, that it consists of associations of individuals linked by a common geography, system of government, and economic ties.

Some of these assumptions are definitive of liberalism, and others are views which tend to go along with it in the context of health care. Together they constitute the bare bones of a coherent philosophy of health care and much besides.

Nevertheless, there are ideas in the contemporary consciousness which lead people to question these assumptions. Out of these ideas a point of view can be developed which challenges classical liberalism. Some of these ideas go back to the Beveridge Report, or earlier to late nineteenth-century 'citizenship' movements (Vincent and Plant 1984). But others spring from new movements of thought on the nature of health and how it should be pursued. All are to be found at least in vague form in contemporary social attitudes, and we shall develop them by means of a critique of liberalism which derives from our conception of citizenship.

10.3 Health as a value

The first assumption of the liberal position on health and health care is that health is not a positive value in its own right, but simply a means to attain other values. Health promotion, particularly in its emphasis on positive health—on being all you can be—must reject the first liberal assumption. But it might be objected that just to assume that health is a value in its own right is simply to express the over-enthusiasm of health promoters. Our book is concerned with basic principles and we must therefore try to *establish* that health is indeed a value in its own right. When that is done it will then be appropriate to consider what sort of value it is.

It will be remembered that we argued that the idea of a value is best approached from the point of view of the activity of valuing. To value something, we said, is to choose it for its own sake in preference to other alternatives. Now, it is not immediately obvious that health fits this account, for two reasons. It might be argued, first, that one does not choose health at all, one either has it or does not have it. And it might be argued, secondly, that even if there is a sense in which one can choose health, it is not chosen for its own sake, but for the sake of the values which cannot be attained without it. This expresses the liberal assumption we are presently discussing.

The first point is valid but not fundamental. It is true that one cannot exactly choose health in the way in which one can choose new clothes. But 'choosing health' is just a shorthand way of speaking of choosing goods and lifestyles which are likely to conduce to or enhance health.

The second point again is valid but not the whole truth. It is valid in that health is certainly an instrumental value, and may be chosen for that reason. This is true whether we are thinking in terms of the individual or of society. To see health in this way is to see it in utilitarian terms. If a society is going to flourish then its members must be healthy. There is therefore a utilitarian justification—a justification in terms of health economics—for a government to promote health. Equally, in the life of the individual, the possession of health is a necessary condition of the attainment of other goods. To describe health as an instrumental value with utilitarian justification is not of course to suggest that it is unimportant. Even if health were simply a means to others' ends it would still be of the first importance, granted that it is a means or a necessary condition for so many other individual and social values. In other words, what we have listed as the first assumption of liberalism about health and health care is correct in its first part.

But there are limitations to this approach to health. First, it depicts health as being good simply for what it brings, whereas it is more plausible to argue that health is also good for what it is. In other words, health is not only an instrumental value, but a value in its own right. Secondly, if health were simply an instrumental value, there would be limits to reasonable governmental promotion of health. In other words, the political justification for promoting health would need to be in terms of preventing ill-health, or promoting functional health in the sense of the ability to carry on a job and not be a drain on resources. But we wish to claim that the government does have a duty to promote health in the positive sense. We must therefore, as a first step, argue that health is a value in its own right. We shall argue for the second step—that health is a value governments should promote—in Section 10.5. How can the case for the first step be made out?

One obvious reason for valuing health for its own sake is that disease, illness, sickness, or disability are likely to be painful or unpleasant, whereas there are positive pleasures, glows of fitness and so on, which accompany the peak of health, and a sense of well-being accompanying more ordinary good health. We have discussed this in Chapter 2. Satisfactions of this kind are values in that they are desired for their own sake.

This argument is acceptable, but its scope is limited since not all forms of the absence of health are painful, even in a wide sense of 'painful' which includes 'uncomfortable' or 'distressing'. Moreover, if health is valued in this way, in terms of pleasure and the absence of pain, it is being regarded merely as a 'liking value', not as something to be approved of and recommended, and as making a reasonable claim on government support. We have seen that health is an instrumental value with social and individual utility, and that it is a 'liking value'. Our question now is whether it can be seen as an ideal or moral value, in such a way that people who cherish health are to be approved of and people who squander it are to be disapproved of. To put it another way, we can refer to Aristotle who distinguished three types of thing which people desire: the useful, the pleasant, and the noble. It is easy to explain, as we have done, how health can be desired under the first two headings and we shall now try to explain how it can be desired under the third, as an ideal value (Downie and Telfer 1980; p. 26).

To see health as an ideal value is to have a biological or purposive idea of how our species is 'meant' to be. There are various ways of explaining this purposive idea. One way might be in terms of a wise and good God whose creative blueprint we should try to exemplify as far as possible, from whom we hold our bodies and minds in trust, and to whom we have a duty to keep them in good repair. It is worth noting, however, that a religious approach to health does not necessarily produce this conclusion. There are some strands in religious thinking in terms of which the body is depicted as evil, and the flesh as something to be mortified rather than preserved. From this point of view, a believer might thank God for his ill-health as something which keeps him from evil. But there is more characteristically a strong strain of the importance of healing the body and mind in religious thought, and that strain provides a religious justification for seeing health as an ideal value.

A second approach might be a secular one in terms of respect for the species; it might be said that it is incumbent on us as human beings to make our human nature flourish. This is an idea which goes back to Plato and has perennial appeal. J. S. Mill (1859; Chapter 3) states it as follows:

Human nature is not a machine to be built after a model, and set to do exactly the work prescribed for it, but a tree, which requires to grow and develop on all sides according to the tendency of the inward forces which make it a living thing.

This passage brings out the biological idea that health as such, apart from its usefulness and its pleasantness, is a value in its own right. The idea is certainly a source of strong feeling in many people, and it is common to hear disapproval of those who are thought to be ruining their health gratuitously.

A third source of the idea that health is a value involves an aesthetic view of health. This view is connected with the biological one, and can be connected also with the religious one. In terms of this approach, health is an ideal design with which we should try to make our bodies conform, and in terms of which aberrations are seen as ugly. People can dislike conditions in themselves and see them as ugly simply because they see them as unhealthy. We discussed this in Chapter 2. A subset of this idea connects health with other qualities which call forth human admiration, such as energy. People are approved of for being like a 'dynamo' and pulsating with energy, although they can also be approved of for being calm where that derives from control rather than passivity. These are mixtures of biological and aesthetic ideas but certainly present health as a positive value. There are then various overlapping ways of describing health in terms of which it can be seen as a value to be approved of, as well as found useful.

10.4 Autonomy and health

Assuming that health is a value in its own right (and that the first assumption of liberalism can therefore be rejected), we shall turn to the second assumption of the liberal position—that people have a right to pursue their own health but no duty to do so unless their ill-health is harming others. This assumption is often thought to be an expression of autonomy interpreted in terms of Mill's 'harm principle' (which we shall shortly discuss). It will emerge that the second assumption can also be challenged.

It might be thought that there is no difficulty about the relationship between autonomy and the pursuit of health within the life or activities of one person. If people pursue health, this is not an impairment or diminution of their autonomy but an expression of it. But can people exercise their autonomy at the *expense* of their own health? If 'exercising autonomy' were simply a matter of doing whatever one wanted, and if health were not a value, then this would be logically possible. But it will be remembered that we have argued that the autonomous person is not simply self-determining but also self-governing, where to be 'self-governing' means to be able to guide one's own conduct in terms of values. Moreover, we have also argued in the previous section of this chapter that health is a value. If follows that if a person knowingly pursues a lifestyle which is destructive of his or her health this cannot count as an expression of autonomy, unless other values are involved. This qualification must be added because a person may knowingly pursue a course of action which will destroy his or her own health, but do so in the service of others. For example, someone may volunteer for service in an unhealthy part of the world, thus endangering personal health for another worthwhile value. Our view is that health is *a* value, not that it is the supreme value. But since it is *a* value it always ought to be one regulator of autonomous behaviour.

More typical problems arise when we note that A's exercise of autonomy may affect B's pursuit of health. The classical liberal solution to this problem is in terms of the 'harm principle'; that A's right to exercise his or her autonomy should be limited if, but only if, he or she is harming B's interests, which in this context is B's health. This is the liberal idea of freedom, 'negative freedom' or freedom from external interference provided one is not harming others. The formulation of this position which is typically quoted here is that of J. S. Mill (*ibid*; Chapter 1):

the sole end for which mankind are warranted, individually or collectively, in interfering with the liberty of action of any of their number, is self-protection . . . His own good, either physical or moral, is not a sufficient warrant.

If we place this liberal principle in the context of health promotion it both gives warrant for the most obvious sorts of health legislation, and also sets limits to paternalistic health care intervention for the patient's 'own good'.

To begin with the second point, the liberal principle is claiming that no doctor or health legislation can justifiably seek to compel people to take steps to protect or improve their health. This liberal right is safeguarded in many ways. For example, people may discharge themselves from hospital, and they must sign a form consenting to an operation, and so on; but of course this right is confined to aspects of their autonomy which affect only their own interests, and, as we shall see, it is a right which does not really extend very far, even within a liberal framework. This takes us back to the first point—the liberal warrant for health legislation.

First of all, and obviously, a person's right to exercise autonomy may be legitimately curtailed by health legislation when he or she is suffering from certain sorts of infectious disease or mental illness such that the interests or health of others are liable to be harmed.

There is no difficulty about the acceptance of this restriction in general terms. The problems arise over the more detailed application of it. For example, a topical question concerns the nature and extent of the restrictions which should be placed on sufferers from AIDS, or the extent of justifiable investigation or reporting of those who may be HIV-positive. Again, it is controversial how far those who are mentally ill should be detained against their will, or what sort of treatment they should have if they are detained.

Pressure for legislation is generated as more becomes known about how diseases are transmitted. For example, the dangers of 'passive smoking' are now appreciated, and other sorts of environmental pollution are now known to cause disease. There is therefore a case for curbing the freedom of both individuals and corporate bodies, such as industries, in the name of the autonomy of other individuals. This issue is, of course, a source of much political debate. Some countries, such as Norway, have banned smoking in many public places, and various 'watchdogs' keep a close eye on the consequences of the operation of the nuclear industry. But, although there can be political debate about applications of the 'preventing harm to others' idea, the general principle is clear and acceptable.

A second issue concerning the way in which a lack of attention to health may affect the autonomy of others turns on the premise that the vast majority of people play some part in the divisions of labour and make a contribution to society. In other words, it is true, and indeed necessarily true, that citizens have social duties; and most people are citizens. But if we fail to perform our social duties, then either someone else has to perform them for us, or other people are in some way harmed or inconvenienced. Either way involves a lessening of some person's autonomy. But we cannot perform our social duties adequately or at all without health. The liberal principle therefore justifies, if not health legislation to force us to be healthy, at least the claim that there are *moral* duties to others to maintain our own health.

A third argument which can be used to justify limiting our autonomy in the interests of the pursuit of health is that health care, under any system, is a scarce resource. Health care used by one person is therefore at the expense of health care available for others.

The argument of this section has been that within a liberal framework there is a right but no duty to pursue our own health, unless by not pursuing our own health we are harming others. We draw attention to the limited extent of the freedom that even this liberal view gives us, because of the way in which we affect each other's interests in society. But in any case we have rejected the liberal position on this and have claimed that health is a value in its own right, and that to be autonomous is to be not just self-determining or entitled to do what we might want, but also self-governing and obliged to regulate our conduct by values, including health. To say this, however, is just to say that there is a *moral* duty to pursue our own health. Does a *government* via health legislation, education, and health campaigns have a duty to safeguard or enhance our health other than to prevent harm? To ask this question is to invite discussion of assumptions 3–5 of the liberal position listed in Section 10.2.

10.5 Government interventions

Has the State any justification for using fiscal policy to promote health, or for passing legislation to promote positive health? This is certainly recommended, as we have seen, by principle 3 of the WHO document quoted on p. 168. But the objection might be that positive health is an *ideal* of the good life rather than a *necessity*, and the State has no duty to promote specific ideals of the good life. This follows from the third assumption of the liberal position listed in Section 10.2.

This objection might be rebutted on the grounds that there is a causal link between the negative sense of health (not being ill) and positive health, such that if the promotion of the conditions conducive to better health in this negative sense can be justified (as it can on any reasonable political theory), then a justification for the promotion of positive health can be found on the same basis. The claim is that the promotion of positive health will bring about physical and mental health states which are resistant or more resistant to disease agents. A claim of this sort would need a great deal of empirical evidence to support it, and in any case is always in danger of being made true by definition—if you do succumb to ill-health then you did not have enough positive health. Nevertheless, at a common sense level it seems obviously true that if you are in general terms fit, then you are less likely to succumb to disease; and if you do succumb to disease, then you will recover more quickly if you enjoy 'positive health'. If, therefore, there is justification for the promotion of health in the negative sense, the same justification holds for the promotion of positive health.

It might be said that this argument depends on an empirical premise—the so-called 'law of disease'—which is hard to establish, however plausible it seems to common sense. It would therefore be preferable if there were some way of arguing that the government does have a duty to promote health in the positive sense as an ideal of the good life.

A stronger and simpler way of arguing that a government does have a duty to promote positive health is to refer to the preamble to the Constitution of WHO (1946), which asserts that there is a right to positive health. In ambitious terms it states: 'The enjoyment of the highest attainable standard of health is one of the fundamental rights of every human being without distinction of race, religion, political belief, economic or social condition.' If this is a fundamental right then presumably there is a correlative duty laid upon governments to implement it. In other words, acceptance of the WHO Constitution commits States to health and welfare policies. How far such policies can be implemented no doubt turns on the wealth of the country, but there can be no doubt that wealthy Western nations are committed to implementing fiscal and legislative policies to enhance positive health. In our next chapter on 'Social Justice' we shall look in more detail at the limits and limitations of State intervention in this area.

To argue that there is a duty on governments to promote health for its own sake still leaves some questions unanswered. Supposing there is such a duty, can it be implemented other than at the expense of individual autonomy? To discuss this question is to examine assumptions 4 and 5 of the liberal position listed in Section 10.2: that health legislation necessarily removes autonomy and that autonomy is simply the absence of constraint.

It is easy to slip into the error of regarding all legislation on the model of the criminal law—as restrictive prohibition backed by sanction. But this is an oversimplified way of looking at some health legislation. For example, legislation may require public bodies to make provision for the disabled. This is more aptly seen as a positive creation of new opportunities than as negative prohibition. Again, there are legal requirements on factory owners to restrict unpleasant pollutants, and on car manufacturers to ensure certain safety standards. Indeed, there is an enormous range of health legislation with a positive slant, and whereas this may diminish the freedom of some groups in society, it certainly extends the freedom of the majority and improves their quality of life.

This now takes us to the fifth assumption of the liberal position, an assumption about the nature of autonomy itself. Is autonomy just the absence of constraint? There is no simple way of answering this question. Any attempt to say 'such and such is the central idea of autonomy' is likely to do violence to some important aspect of it. It is possible, however, to distinguish at least one positive aspect to the concept. Just as we distinguished a negative side to health as the absence of disease, and a positive side embracing well-being, so it is possible to distinguish a negative side to autonomy as the absence of constraint, and a positive side as 'being empowered' or as 'self-determination'.

If we think of autonomy in this way then health legislation is not *removing* our individual autonomy but rather *enhancing* it. In improving the general quality of life, legislation can add to our autonomy. This is obviously the case if we consider the example of provision for the disabled, but it is true also of anti-pollution legislation, and many other types of health legislation.

We shall, in conclusion, pull together the main threads of the argument. We have been addressing two main questions: what is the relationship between the pursuit of health and the exercise of autonomy; and what ought to be the position of a government on the pursuit of health by its subjects? In discussing these questions we have considered the liberal framework of thinking on health autonomy and politics, and the ways in which the ideas of health promotion modify that framework.

Taking the first question, we noted that, in terms of liberal assumptions, individuals may exercise their autonomy in the pursuit of health but are not obliged to do so because health is seen as an instrumental value enabling its possessor to obtain a wide range of other goods. Health is thereby simply a causal factor in the pursuit of the good life or, at best, what we have termed a 'liking value'. From the health promotion point of view, however, health is not just an external instrumental means to the exercise of autonomy but an internal component means. Positive health is not just a necessary condition of self-realization but is an actual realization of the self. This last point is difficult and needs some further explanation.

The liberal, we said, sees health as an instrumental means to realizing other sorts of value, but does not see it as itself a value. In the same way, the scaffolding, lorries, cement mixers, building tools, etc. are external instrumental means to the building of a house, and they have no value in their own right. But the bricks, glass, wood, and slates are internal component means to the house; they are part of the finished product. In a similar way, we are claiming that positive health is not just an external instrumental means to the good life for human beings; it is a component value, a part of the good life.

Turning now to the question of how far the government is obliged or justified in using fiscal policy and health legislation to further the positive health of individuals and enhance their autonomy, we argued that if there is a causal link between furthering positive health and preventing ill-health, then there is a duty on governments to further the positive health of individuals as a means of preventing ill-health. More strongly we argued that to the extent that governments accept the WHO Constitution, which states that there is a right possessed by individuals to the best possible health, there is a correlative duty on governments to do what they can to improve health.

Two important qualifications should be noted about this justification. The first is that it does not follow from the fact that there is a human right to health and a correlative duty on governments to do what they can to improve health that there is not also a moral duty on people to do what they can to improve their own health. The parallel is with education. Governments have a duty to create facilities for education, but people have a duty to make the best use of these facilities.

The second qualification is that the duty of a government to improve the health status of its citizens cannot be separated from the duties of social justice. Many studies have shown that the major threats to health in this country are not evenly distributed across the population but are heavily concentrated in the lower social classes. The main thrust of health promotion should therefore be in this area, and again there are parallels with education. It is to the problem of social justice that we shall next turn. The discussion of this problem will also enable us to examine the final assumption of the liberal position—that 'society' is just a fiction to refer to assemblages of individuals and their individual responsibilities.

10.6 Conclusions

1. Health promotion is strongly normative; it endeavours to persuade people to adopt certain lifestyles, and is committed to furthering certain values.
2. The prevailing assumptions of Western society are those of liberalism, and health promotion (which arises from certain new currents of thought) leads to the modification or even rejection of certain of these assumptions.
3. In particular, health promotion sees health not just as an instrumental and 'liking' value (although it is these) but also as an ideal or moral value, something to be approved of for its own sake.
4. Since to be autonomous is not just to be self-determining or free to do what one wants, but also to be self-governing or subject to values, people have a moral duty to pursue health for its own sake, as a value, and not just to prevent harm to others (although even that considerably limits their freedom).
5. But in pursuing health in the fullest sense for its own sake people are expressing their autonomy, their true selves.
6. The government has a duty via health legislation, fiscal policy, and other means to enhance the positive health of individuals since this follows from the WHO claim that there is a human right to health in the fullest sense.
7. Health legislation and fiscal policy do not diminish autonomy but enhance it.

11 Justice, health, and society

It is not immediately clear that questions of social justice are raised by health and its distribution, as distinct from health care, health determinants, and their distribution. Moreover, even if we suppose that questions of social justice do arise over health, we must not immediately conclude that it is entirely the fault of a government if there is social injustice, or even that social injustice in health, if it exists, can always be rectified by government intervention. The relationships between these ideas of health, health care, health determinants, and social justice are of importance to health promotion, since a clarification will help to clarify the political stance of health promotion. Our argument will be that the political stance of health promotion derives from its own professional concerns.

11.1 Health, health care, and health determinants

Is health not just a brute fact about people? For example, it is just a brute fact that some people have the natural capacity to run faster than others, or have better brains than others, or are more attractive than others. This may be unfortunate, but it is not a question of justice, unless we think that God has been unfair. So why is the same not true of health? It might, of course, be said that people have a certain room for choice in respect of their natural capacities—they can improve or neglect their natural capacities and might be praised or blamed for so doing. And again the same is true of health; people can to a limited extent take steps which improve or destroy their health and we might praise or blame them. But these considerations, even if they bring health within the sphere of morality (see Section 10.4), do not make it a matter of social justice. So is health a matter of social justice, or is it just misleading to think of it in those terms?

It might be said that at least *health care* is a matter of social justice. For example, if it could be shown that for no good reason the distribution of GPs, hospitals, and ancillary services was uneven, then this fact would be a legitimate cause of complaint to a government. Even this point assumes what some liberal purists would deny, that it is the duty of a government, as distinct from the market, to concern itself with the distribution of health care. But despite this qualification there is obviously a case for discussing the distribution of health care in the language of justice.

Moreover, *health determinants* also seem to lie within the field of social justice. By 'health determinants' we mean all those factors, such as housing, diet, leisure facilities, which influence health status. Once again, some theorists might argue that those commodities are market-related and do not directly raise questions of social justice. But most Western governments have diluted the purity of market-based liberalism with welfarist ideas, and in so far as governments, local or national, provide or regulate the supply of such health determinants, then they may be discussed in the language of social justice.

So far, then, we have distinguished health, health care, and health determinants, and have maintained that, whereas health falls only marginally within the sphere of social justice, health care and health determinants are largely matters of social justice (the extent depending on the extent to which the purity of market-based liberalism is diluted with welfarist elements).

Unfortunately, however, this account of the relationship between these concepts is too simple. According to the models of health and health promotion recommended in this book, the concepts of health, health care, and health determinants are closely connected, and therefore the connection of each with justice is closer than emerges on our account so far, as we shall now show.

First, there is an obvious link between health and health care, in that where the health of a given population compares poorly with that of a wider population there is a *prima facie* case for investigating the adequacy of the health care provided. Secondly, there is also a close causal link between health determinants and individual health, in that such matters as damp housing are obviously factors in producing poor health states in individuals. Indeed, that is why they are called 'health determinants'. This point suggests that, thirdly, and more controversially, the link between health and health determinants is also *conceptual*: health is not just a property of individuals but of social relationships and social structures. This claim requires some expansion.

We have argued that persons are essentially social; it is their nature to be citizens (Section 9.5). Their positive health is therefore continuous with the quality of their social relationships and structures. This is implicit in the WHO definition of health from which we began in Chapter 2. But 'social relationships' and 'social structures' are simply grand terms for what are normally regarded as health determinants—housing, employment, leisure and cultural facilities. In other words, the distinction between health and health determinants is by no means clear-cut, and we can speak of health as being experienced through social relationships. Indeed, we speak quite naturally, and not metaphorically, when we say that the atmosphere in a school, or even more generally in a community, is one of well-being. Perhaps this point is most dramatically made in the example of a well-run and humanely administered hospice. We can say of it that well-being pervades its atmosphere—it enables its inmates to live until they die—regardless of the fact that its inmates, from the point of view of negative health, are terminally ill. In such an institution the social relationships and social structures can properly be said to express well-being (see Section 2.3).

Fourthly, the connection between health care and health determinants is not sharp. Thus, it is by no means clear whether such matters as the provision of community centres for the elderly, or equipment, toilet facilities, and accessible buildings for the disabled, are health care or health determinants. And what of meals-on-wheels, nursery facilities, rehabilitation centres for alcoholics or for mentally disturbed people?

If, then, it is possible to maintain that there are these close connections between health, health care, and health determinants, and if it is plausible to maintain that the latter two raise questions of social justice, then we can also maintain that health itself raises questions of social justice. It does not, of course, follow that it is the fault of the government if a society is unhealthy and unjust. It is common but superficial to heap all the blame for social injustice on the government of the day, and we shall discuss the role of government intervention in Sections 11.3 and 11.4. But the immediate requirement for the argument is to analyse the concept of social justice as it affects health, health care, and health determinants.

11.2 Social justice

The discussion of social justice in health care is often put in the language of equality and we shall discuss it in that language. The very general ideal behind the National Health Service, and other systems that have similar ideals, is that each person has a right to *equal consideration* in respect of health care and that it is the duty of the State to observe that right.

This notion of 'equal consideration', however, needs considerably more examination (Downie and Telfer 1980). In some contexts the demand for equal consideration is merely a demand for consistent treatment as between one person and another: in other words, a demand that people be treated in accordance with some rule which can be formulated. This demand for consistency seems to clash with the more personalized aspects of case-work or patient care, which stress the impossibility of general rules and the uniqueness of the individual situation. But where benefits are being distributed, clients and patients are keen to demand consistency ('Why won't you give to me what you gave to him?') and regard as unfair any difference of this kind which seems to be an arbitrary exception. Consistency is an important aspect of social justice in the context of discussion of the distribution of ill-health among different social classes and geographical areas. Consistency, then, is necessary if distribution of benefit (and, of course, health education, medical treatment, and social work services are themselves benefits) is to be seen as fair.

But consistency alone is not sufficient for fairness. A principle of distribution which could be applied consistently, such as 'Never spend time on an alcoholic', might itself be unfair. To get nearer to the moral principle of equal consideration, we need to find some way of ruling out such possibilities.

What is required is that all differences of treatment be based on a criterion which group like cases together, and distinguish unlike cases, for morally appropriate reasons. In this context the obvious criterion is *need*. Since the aim of proffering help is to meet needs, those whose need is greatest should get more help than those whose need is less, and those whose need is equal should get equal help. This principle, of justified differences in treatment based on the criterion of differing degrees of need, is neatly illustrated by those benefits which are scaled according to the size of the family which is to receive them, or by the provision of more repeat consultations to people of lower social classes to compensate for lack of coping skills (Whitehead 1987).

We shall call this requirement, that any differences of treatment be based on morally appropriate reasons, a principle of equity. Equity is not the same as consistency since it says not only that like cases must be treated equally but also that unlike cases must be treated unequally. In other words, equity can be expressed in 'positive discrimination' (see Section 4.5). As we have seen, equity presupposes a criterion for justifiable differences in the way people are treated. In the context of health this will normally be need. Of course, in other contexts, such as education, other criteria might be relevant, such as capacity, but we shall stick to the health context and the criterion based on need.

Since the term 'need' is frequently used in discussions of social welfare, including health promotion, it may be helpful to offer a brief analysis of it. The basic idea in all uses of the term 'need' is that of a necessary condition for the bringing about of an objective. For example, someone might need pen and paper in order to write a letter, or need to train in order to stay in the team. To approach the question from another angle, we can always ask the person who claims to need something, 'What do you need it for?' and the answer will specify an objective. This basic sense of 'need' is value-neutral: we might need a crow bar to break into the safe.

There is, however, a specialized sense of the basic idea of need which is not value-neutral. We use the term 'needs' to refer to the goods and services which it is rational to want as the necessary conditions of a given level of welfare. Needs in this specialized sense often refer to social service benefits including health care and health promotion benefits. Thus to say that one social group has greater needs (for health promotion, or similar benefits) than others is to say that these benefits are among the conditions necessary to raise them to a specified level of health or welfare. It should be clear from this analysis of the concept why 'need' is the criterion generally applied in contexts of health inequalities.

So far, then, we have looked at two senses of the right to equal consideration which makes up the concept of social justice in a health context. These were consistency of treatment, a principle which is necessary but not sufficient for social justice in health care, and equity—equality of treatment based on need. Are these concepts sufficient to express our intuitions of social justice?

Perhaps, but some thinkers would have reservations about the adequacy of equity on the grounds that it is both *derivative*, in that it depends on another value, such as need or capacity, before it comes into operation; and *relative*, in that it involves equality only with others in the same group, not with everyone. There is, however, a third approach to 'equal consideration' which we may call *egalitarian equality*. The third sense seems to be neither derivative nor relative; it advocates that all people be treated equally for equality's sake, not just in the course of pursuing other values. A principle of egalitarian equality entails not only trying, when serving people's needs, to do so in an equitable manner, but also redistributing benefits simply to make people more equal when need is not in question. In practice, of course, this distinction between equity and egalitarianism is not clear-cut. What one group sees as organizing taxation and benefits in an equitable way proportionate to the needs of all concerned, another group sees as 'the egalitarian politics of envy'. Again, what can be construed in a given society as needed depends in part on an egalitarian consideration, viz., what other people have: in a society where most people have television, a mains water supply is not a luxury but a need. This point is made in the Black Report (1980; p. 107) as follows:

Poverty is also a relative concept, and those who are unable to share the amenities or facilities provided within a rich society, or who are unable to fulfil the social and occupational obligations placed upon them by virtue of their limited resources, can properly be regarded as poor. They may also be relatively disadvantaged in relation to the risks of illness or accident or the factors positively promoting health.

The spirit of egalitarian equality is important for the present argument, since it lies behind the Black Report and many discussions of social justice in the context of health, health care, and health determinants.

We spoke just now of the egalitarians' aim to 'make people more equal'. But the question immediately arises—equal in what respect? For it is possible to draw a broad contrast between the ideal of equality in respect of opportunity—equality in the starting and running conditions of the race of life—and equality in respect of outcome—the ideal of proceeding side by side throughout the race to a 'tie' at the finish. It is fairly common for those of moderate opinion to commit themselves to the first of these ideals rather than the second. But the second also is aimed at by many social thinkers at the present time. Moreover, the truth may be (although believers in equality of opportunity have not always faced up to it) that the first cannot be secured in independence of the second. For even if you provide equality of opportunity, then, granted the truth of some uncontroversial propositions about the variation in human ability, industry, etc., the tendency will be towards inequality of outcome or satisfaction. Perhaps, then, we must say that if the welfare services are really concerned with equality as an ideal, they are concerned to secure not just 'equal opportunities' but 'equal outcomes'. In other words, there is commitment to positive discrimination. This seems to be the view of the Black Report.

To bring this out, consider an argument in the Black Report concerned with equality of opportunity of access to GP consultations. They point out that for most years covered by the General Household Survey the number of people consulting a doctor, and the average number of consultations, has tended to increase with descending social class. In other words, the figures seem to suggest that, for curative if not preventive services, there is equality of opportunity to use the services. But the Black Report (p. 69) does not draw this conclusion. The authors say: 'This may partially miss the point. It may be that the proper basis for comparing rates of consultation is not one of simple population but of the *need* for care'. In other words, they conclude that the greater consultation rates suggest a greater need for care which is not being satisfied. The preferred ideal is therefore thought to be equality of outcome or satisfaction, and not just equality of opportunity.

The same point is made by Whitehead (1987; p. 271). One study cited suggested that doctors gave more repeat consultations to lower social class patients to compensate for their lack of coping skills. This suggests equality of opportunity. Another study took the same data to suggest that 'the lower occupational classes had more illness which was life-threatening and more painful in nature than higher classes'. In other words, the second writer did not see equality of outcome because there is lack of equality of need.

So far we have considered three applications of the moral idea of equality of consideration: the equality of consistency; the relative equality of equity which derives from need; egalitarian equality which is neither derivative nor relative.

All three notions of equality, however, presuppose a fourth more fundamental kind of equality in terms of which it is assumed that all human beings ought to be regarded as equal. Egalitarian equality assumes that *all* human beings ought to have equal satisfactions, and does not exclude any group from its scope. Equity, although it does not say that everyone should be treated equally, incorporates the demand that differences in treatment must be *morally justified*: in other words, the presumption is that people should be treated equally *unless* there is moral warrant for treating them differently. Both principles therefore rule out the option of leaving some group out of one's moral calculations altogether. Thus, respect for equity precludes us from saying 'Don't bother about the mentally handicapped', for instance.

But if the underlying concept is supposed to involve the notion that there is a respect in which people *are* equal, as a matter of fact, it is clearly mistaken. People are manifestly *unequal* in physique, in mental capacity, in physical attractiveness, in moral goodness, in any respect that can be thought of. We do however speak of people as of equal *worth* or *value*. Given that people are *not* in fact equal, can any sense be made of this idea?

The notion of human beings as of equal worth makes sense if it is regarded, not as a statement of fact about human beings, but as a principle prescribing how they are to be treated. But the importance of the principle does not lie in its stress on *equality*, but in its stress on human worth. The point is that each individual human being is to be treated as having worth or value in him- or herself. Human beings do not have a price—they are not replaceable by anything else, even by other human beings—they individually have what Kant calls *dignity*, the value of something which is irreplaceable. This is again the principle of respect for the individual which we have already introduced (Section 9.6), and it carries with it the idea that no one's claims may be ignored, however great the gain to others, because a price cannot be put on any individual's welfare. This point can be put in terms of equality by saying that everyone is of equal importance, but the equality is after all *derivative*, in the sense that it depends on another moral value, that of respect for the individual. We can depict consistency, equity, and egalitarian equality as manifestations of respect for the individual, deployed in a social context; all three, but particularly egalitarian equality, are also called social justice, and all three are constitutive of societal well-being, or a flourishing society.

11.3 Explaining the health divide

The preceding discussion of the complex idea of equality has brought out that whether we stress consistency, equity, or egalitarian equality, large inequalities in health status are morally unjustifiable. Does the fact that there are wide differences in health status among social classes therefore constitute an *injustice*? The answer here depends on the explanation of the health inequalities between the social classes. The Black Report (1980) and its sequel *The health divide* (Whitehead 1987) offer four possible explanations of the differentials. The first of these is what they call the 'artefact' explanation—that the method of measuring occupational class artificially inflates the size and importance of health differences. This is rightly dismissed on the grounds, among others, that on any index of social circumstances the findings are more or less consistent with those based on occupational class gradients.

The second explanation is in terms of natural and social selection. People in poor health slide down the occupational and social scales. There is something in this but the evidence suggests that it accounts for only a small proportion of the health differential between social classes.

The third explanation, the structuralist–materialist explanation, stresses the conditions and pressures of the environment—poor housing, dangerous work, fewer resources—which lead to poor health states.

The fourth explanation stresses cultural–behavioural differences; lower social classes adopt a more dangerous and health-damaging lifestyle than higher social classes, as a result of a 'culture of poverty' or 'transmitted deprivation'.

Clearly, the most plausible explanations, which are all elaborated with sophistication in the Black Report and *The health divide*, are the third and fourth, and each of them appeals to a different set of values. The fourth explanation stresses individual moral responsibility for health states. It might be said that nobody can now be ignorant of the dangers of cigarette smoking or of a high-fat diet. If, therefore, people persist in both, their consequential ill-health is their own fault. By contrast, the third explanation depicts behaviour as determined by social and economic conditions. A good example of the differences in approach is in the rival explanations of childhood accidents (Whitehead 1987; p. 62).

The observation that children from lower social groups have more accidents than children from higher groups may be explained by the behavioural view as due to more reckless risk-taking behaviour in this group and inadequate care by parents. The materialist view would highlight the unsafe play areas, the lack of fenced-off gardens, and the greater difficulty of supervising children's play from high-rise housing. In the latter view the environment is dictating the behaviour of both mother and child.

What bearing do these rival explanations have on the question of whether the health divide constitutes a social injustice? If the fourth explanation is stressed, then it is arguable that the health divide is not mainly a matter of social injustice. There may be some social injustice if it can be shown that people belonging to lower social classes are not adequately informed, or that health care, housing, and leisure facilities are sub-standard. But basically this approach emphasizes individual responsibility for poor health in lower social classes. Many writers on health promotion use the term 'victim-blaming' to describe this emphasis (see p. 31), and no doubt it is sometimes no more than that.

But, as we shall see, there is also an important and valid point to be made through this approach: health cannot be achieved through any 'top-down' services or hand-outs, but only via a 'bottom-up' approach. Any other view is basically patronizing to the people involved. Autonomy, of course, as we have already stressed, is something to be *achieved*, rather than something which people possess regardless of their social and economic conditions, and it is this that the third explanation emphasizes; the term 'empowerment' brings this out. Hence, as we have stressed, many writers on health promotion prefer to use that term rather than 'autonomy'.

Does it then constitute a social injustice that health determinants, the social and economic conditions for health, are much poorer in some than in other areas of society? It may do, but no one should underestimate the consequences, economic and political, of attempting to remedy this state of affairs. When the Black Report was published in 1980 the Secretary of State for Social Services pointed out in a Foreword that the additional expenditure involved in endorsing the recommendations was upward of £2 billion per year at 1980 prices. He therefore did not endorse the recommendations. Now it is easy to blame governments for failing to improve social conditions, and the evidence is that the health divide has increased since 1980. But in a democratic society a government can do only what its electorate shows a political will for it to do, and there is no evidence that the electorate is willing to countenance the massive redistribution of resources which would be involved in an additional expenditure of that magnitude. To say this is not to say that much more cannot be done by governments even within this democratic mandate.

Indeed, even in terms of a liberal view, a government can still be pressed to do a great deal towards creating a healthy environment, insisting on regulations for industrial waste, the minimizing of pollution, and so on. The argument is that even on a negative conception of government there would be a requirement to protect citizens from disease, and no clear line can be drawn between this and the positive furthering of the health of the inhabitants by public health legislation. It is important to stress this because it is common to despise *laissez-faire* political philosophy on the grounds, among others, that is has nothing positive to advocate on health care. Yet if it can consistently advocate public health legislation it can, and historically did, achieve as much an improvement in the nation's health as the National Health Service; for an adequate system of sanitation and other population health protection measures have done more for the health of the nation than any subsequent improvements in medical services, including the present high-cost technological medicine. But there is no political will in Western democracies for the massive redistribution entailed by the Black Report.

Let us turn from health determinants to the provision of health care facilities and services for individuals. The question is whether they can be categorized, in liberal terms, in the same way as population health measures. In other words, can the provision of health care by the State be seen as the provision of a commodity which is under-supplied in market terms and one which therefore makes a claim on a liberal government?

On a pure version of the liberal or *laissez-faire* theory of the State, health service would not count as what economists call 'joint' or 'non-excludable' or 'under-supplied' in market terms. They would not therefore call for government action, and therefore inequality in the distribution of those goods would not constitute a social injustice, as distinct from an individual failing to ensure adequate health insurance. But most countries in the West, apart perhaps from the USA, do not have pure versions of liberal individualism, and in diluted forms of liberalism the state provision of health care does not seem anomalous.

Now, if the state does provide health care it can reasonably be criticized for any wide differences in the distribution of health care, and this will be a criticism in the language of social justice. It is a matter for complex factual investigation, such as is exemplified in the Black Report and *The health divide*, whether any given countries can be criticized for this at any given period. We shall not dwell on this, important though it is, because many studies have dealt with it. It is sufficient for us to note the conclusion that on all except pure versions of the liberal state the distribution of health care facilities does raise a question of social justice.

We wish to lay stress on another aspect of the matter. This aspect is still in a sense political, but it raises practical issues which can be taken up by the health promotion movement.

11.4 Community and citizenship

Let us begin by asking the question: 'Suppose a government were to endorse the recommendations of the Black Report, would they bring about health for all?' The answer is 'no', because no amount of improvement in social conditions is a substitute for people themselves taking responsibility for their own health and their own neighbourhood. This is the truth in the cultural/behavioural explanations of the health divide in the Black Report and *The health divide*. On the other hand, it is entirely unrealistic to expect individuals on their own, in deprived areas or circumstances, to take full responsibility for their own health and well-being. Assistance, advice, and leadership are required, and it is precisely this that the health promotion movement is about, and it is from this purely professional concern that the distinctive health promotion concept of 'empowerment' derives.

The provision of professional help in community development (see p. 44) is best carried out on a multi-disciplinary basis. For example, health education/ promotion officers must work along with social work services, local churches, and the general public. The danger to be avoided is the one into which the delivery of health care has fallen. The delivery of health care has often been criticized for using 'top-down' methods and over-emphasizing 'magic bullets', which are wrongly thought by the public to be capable of curing every ailment known to human beings. This criticism, which has been given its most trenchant formulation by Ivan Illich (1977), is that health care workers, and the whole context of health care, have become what we might term 'over-professionalized'. The impression has been conveyed over several decades that an ordinary person cannot really manage his or her own health and welfare, and that for any of the ills of life there is an expert who will help.

There are three connected aspects of this criticism (Downie and Telfer 1980). The first is what we might call the medicalization of ordinary experience. In other words, we have all been encouraged to think that every human anxiety, discomfort, or misery is a medical or related problem. Where in the past people might have thought that sleeplessness is something that you can treat yourself, that anxiety or grief are to be shared with a clergyman, a friend, or a neighbour, or that discomforts or miseries are to be put up with until they go away, we now turn to the doctor for a pill.

Going along with the medicalization of experience there is, secondly, the complementary belief that for every ailment there is an expert to help. Those in the health care business have not discouraged either of these beliefs and have warned of the dangers of not consulting the doctor in time, of not contacting welfare services, of not having regular checks on one's teeth, and so on; and now specialist health promoters have emerged as a new generation of experts dominating the media with the high-pressure selling of positive health.

The outcome of this takes us to the third and most important point for present purposes. The medicalization of ordinary experience plus the rise of the expert has had the result that people have lost confidence in their own abilities to take responsibility for their own health in particular and their own lives in general. Ordinary people have come to feel that they do not have the expertise needed to help with family or similar difficulties. As a consequence many people have lost the feeling that there is a moral need to have any concern for one's neighbour; 'they' can now be relied on to do everything. All three criticisms point in the same direction: the delivery of health care has had a tendency to sap individual freedom, positively conceived, by removing our sense that we are in control of our own health.

The cure for all these ills is the same. Those involved in health care and health promotion must abandon their professional isolation and begin to work *through* the community rather than *on* it, in order to do things *with* the community rather than *to* it. To be fair, there are many signs that this has begun to happen and the health promotion movement can take some credit for the greater stress on *community* involvement in health. There has, in fact, been a growth in recent years of self-help groups—from the familiar Alcoholics Anonymous groups to the many types of parents' groups concerned with education, bereavement, and every sort of serious childhood disease. The growth of such self-help movements should be encouraged and informed by those in professional health care. One of the five principles identified by WHO (1984) is that 'health promotion aims particularly at effective and concrete public participation.'

Indeed, for adequate health care, for the reduction of negative health and the promotion of positive health, we require not just that we should be served by authorized representatives, with the rights, duties, skills, and values of the health care professions; not just that these representatives should co-operate in teams for our total health; for wholeness or well-being we require that we should all see ourselves as members of a collectively responsible society. In other words, the members of the health care professions must be assisted by our own striving to become (in the words of St Paul) members one of another. This view of society depicts it as a community with a communal good not entirely reducible to the individual goods of the persons who make it up. In other words, it is a view of society which is importantly different from the liberal view. It is one alternative to the final liberal assumption (see list in Section 10.2) that 'society' is just a convenient fiction to refer to the individuals who occupy a given area at a given time. To put it another way, if society is just individuals then these individuals are *citizens*, or individuals with social responsibilities and a social well-being. This is one implication of the theory of health education we developed in Section 3.4.

To the extent that there is exclusive emphasis on the *State* delivery of health care to individuals, there is the invitation to see health as a commodity to be supplied by the State. The same is true if we think of health as a commodity bought by private health insurance. But health is not in any sense a commodity. Health and well-being are in the end a set of relationships among citizens. As Beauchamp (1987; p. 72) put it:

Collective goods are ultimately a set of relationships among the citizens of a community, relationships in which the community as a whole participates to obtain desired benefits. These collective goods include aggregate states of welfare or wellbeing, including declining rates of disease and premature deaths; efforts to limit the resources society devotes to personal health services; shared and common access to a good like medical care to foster the sense of community and membership in the group itself. And finally, there are those highly important collective goods, shared or common beliefs and values.

It is clear that we can add a legal system to Beauchamp's list, and in particular one designed to stimulate social responsibility. Indeed, it is plausible to suggest that the increasing government intervention on drunk-driving issues has encouraged a greater social awareness about the dangers of alcohol more generally, and thus a greater sense of community and individual responsibility. In a similar way, legislation designed to assist disabled or handicapped persons can also increase a sense of community responsibility for those groups. In other words, in so far as health legislation and other governmental health policies are directed at increasing community awareness, as distinct from being directed at the good of specific individuals, it is not paternalistic.

We shall conclude by putting out point in terms of grammar, as a change from the more usual sociological or medical models of health and health education. Health can be and traditionally was seen as an *adjective*—a kind of attribute or property which individuals could possess, which could be protected by vaccination and impaired by disease. According to more recent ways of looking at health, health is an *adverb*—a style of living, a way of qualifying the active verbs of living. This is part of the promotional or lifestyle approach to health. But we want to suggest that health can also be seen as a *relational predicate*—that health, especially positive health or well-being, can be seen as a set of relationships in which the community as a whole participate to obtain mutual benefits, benefits which include a decline in ill-health and the enhancement of well-being through the shared values of citizenship.

11.5 Conclusions

1. We argued that the initially plausible view—that health care and health determinants, but not health itself, are appropriate subjects

for judgements of justice—breaks down when the links between all three are noted.

2. Social justice can be understood as (a) consistency in the supply of goods and services to different areas or social classes; (b) equity based on the criterion of need; (c) egalitarianism, or equality for its own sake. Strands (b) and (c) are often confused, and all three presuppose (d) the equality of human worth, which is an expression of the basic principle of respect for the autonomous individual.

3. The difficulties of achieving equity, far less egalitarian equality, are considerable, and although even a market-based government can be expected to show some positive discrimination to affect the balance of social justice, there is no sign that any Western democracy has the political will to make the massive redistribution involved in recommendations such as those of the Black Report.

4. In any case, a 'top-down' governmental intervention cannot bring about health for all in the WHO sense of health. What is needed is a new sense of community responsibility or citizenship. The health promotion movement is essential in facilitating this development.

5. It is in the facilitating of the sense of community by all methods that the political stance of health promotion is to be found.

Further reading

Chapter 2

Aggleton, P. (1990). *Health*. Routledge, London.
Seedhouse, D. (1986). *Health: the foundations for achievement*. Wiley, Chichester.

Chapter 3

Ewles, L. and Simnett, I. (1992). *Promoting health. A practical guide*, (2nd edn). Scutari, London.
Fletcher, C. (1973). *Communication in medicine*. Nuffield Provincial Hospitals Trust, London.

Chapter 4

Ashton, J. and Seymour, H. (1988). *The new public health*. Open University Press, Milton Keynes.
Department of Health and Social Security (1976). *Prevention and health: everybody's business*. HMSO, London.
Faculty of Community Medicine (1986). *Health for all by the year 2000. Charter for action*. Faculty of Community Medicine, London.
Gray, J. A. M. and Fowler, G. (1984). *Essentials of preventive medicine*. Blackwell, Oxford.
Holland, W. W. and Stewart, S. (1990). *Screening in health care* Nuffield Provincial Hospitals Trust, London.
O'Neill, P. (1983). *Health crisis 2000*. World Health Organization, Copenhagen.
Research Unit in Health and Behavioural Change, University of Edinburgh (1989). *Changing the public health*. Wiley, Chichester.
Smith, A. and Jacobson, B. (ed.) (1991). *The nation's health. A strategy for the 1990s*, (revised edn). King Edward's Hospital Fund for London.

Taylor, P. (1985). *The smoke ring: tobacco, money and multinational politics*. Sphere, London.

Chapter 6

Council of Europe Committee of Ministers (1988). *School health education and the role of training of teachers*. Recommendation No. R (88) 7.
David, K. and Williams, T. (ed.) (1987). *Health education in schools*, (2nd edn). Harper and Row, Cambridge.
Department of Education and Science (1977). *Health education in schools*. HMSO, London.
Faculty of Public Health Medicine (1993). *Strategies for health promotion in primary health care*. Faculty of Public Health Medicine, London.
Fowler, G., Gray, M., and Anderson, p. (1993). *Prevention in General Practice*, (2nd edn). Oxford University Press.
Tannahill, A. (1995). *Putting health promotion into primary care strategies*. *Health Bulletin*, **53**, 192–5.

Chapter 9

Beauchamp, T. L. and Childress, J. F. (1993). *Principles of biomedical ethics*, (4th edn). Oxford University Press.
Downie, R. S. and Telfer, E. (1980). *Caring and curing*. Methuen, London.

Chapter 10

Doxiadis, S. (ed.) (1987). *Ethical dilemmas in health promotion*. Wiley, Chichester.
Doxiadis, S. (ed.) (1990). *Ethics in health education*. Wiley, Chichester.

Chapter 11

Campbell, A. V. (1976). *Medicine, health and justice*. Churchill Livingstone, Edinburgh.
Daniels, N. (1985). *Just health care*. Cambridge University Press.
Plant, R., Lesser, H., and Taylor-Gooby, P. (1980). *Political*

philosophy and social welfare. Routledge and Kegan Paul, London.

Vincent, A. and Plant, R. (1984). *Philosophy, politics and citizenship*. Blackwell, Oxford.

References

Ad Hoc Group on Screening (1992). *Report to the health services and public health research board*. Medical Research Council, London.

Ajzen, I. and Fishbein, M. (1977). Attitude–behaviour relations: a theoretical analysis and review of empirical research. *Psychological Bulletin*, **84**, 888–918.

Alderson, M. (1976). *An introduction to epidemiology*, p. 172. Macmillan, London.

Anonymous (1981). Commentary from Westminster. Blocking of Bill on tobacco advertising. *Lancet*, **1**, 1377–8.

Anonymous (1993). The Scottish health strategy. *Health Bulletin*, **51**, 272–5.

Antonovsky, A. (1984). The sense of coherence as a determinant of health. In *Behavioural health. A handbook of health enhancement and disease prevention*, (ed. J. D. Matarrazzo, S. M. Veiss, A. J. Herd, and N. Miller). Wiley, New York.

Antonovsky, A. (1987). *Unravelling the mystery of health*. Jossey Bass, San Francisco.

Arnold, M. F. (1972). Evaluation: a parallel process to planning. In *Administering health systems: issues and perspectives*, (ed. M. F. Arnold, L. V. Blenkenship, and J. M. Hess). Aldine-Atherton, Chicago.

ASH (Action on Smoking and Health), BMA (British Medical Association), and HEA (Health Education Authority) (1988). *Two good reasons for a tobacco pricing policy*. ASH/BMA/HEA, London.

Atkinson, A. B. and Townsend, J. L. (1977). Economic aspects of reduced smoking. *Lancet*, **2**, 492–4.

Baric, L. (1980). Evaluation: obstacles and potentialities. *International Journal of Health Education*, **23**, 142–9.

Beauchamp, D. (1987). Life-style, public health and paternalism. In *Ethical dilemmas in health promotion*, (ed. S. Doxiadis). Wiley, Chichester.

Becker, M. H. (1974). The health belief model and personal health behaviour. *Health Education Monographs*, **2** (4).

Black Report (1980). Published in 1988 as *Inequalities in health*. (ed. P. Townsend, N. Davidson, and M. Whitehead). Penguin, Harmondsworth.

BMA (British Medical Association) (1986). *Smoking out the barons: the campaign against the tobacco industry*. Wiley, Chichester.

Bowling, A. (1991). *Measuring health. A review of quality of life measurement scales*. Open University Press, Milton Keynes.

Cameron, D. (1985). Warning against US tobacco sachets. *The Scotsman*, 26 July.

Catford, J. C. (1983). Positive health indicators—towards a new information base for health promotion. *Community Medicine*, **5**, 125–32.

Chaiken, S. and Stangor, C. (1987). Attitudes and attitude change. *Annual Review of Psychology*, **38**, 575–630.

Chambers, L. W., Sackett, D. L., Goldsmith, C. H., Macpherson, A. S., and McAuley, R. G. (1976). Development and application of an index of social function. *Health Services Research*, **11**, 430–41.

Chisholm, J. W. (1990). The 1990 contract: its history and its content. *British Medical Journal*, **300**, 853–6.

Coopersmith, S. (1967). *The antecedents of self-esteem*. W. H. Freeman, San Francisco.

Cribb, A. (1986). Politics and health in the school curriculum. In *The politics of health education—raising the issues*, (ed. S. Rodmell and A. Watt). Routledge and Kegan Paul, London.

Currie, C. and Todd, J. (1992). *Health behaviours of Scottish schoolchildren: report 1: national and regional patterns*. Health Education Board for Scotland/Research Unit in Health and Behavioural Change, University of Edinburgh, Edinburgh.

Dennis, J., Draper, P., Holland, S., Shipster, P., Speller, V., and Sunter, J. (1982). Prevention is possible if you try. *The Health Services*, **37**, 13.

Department of Health (1991). *The health of the nation. A consultative document for health in England*. HMSO, London.

Department of Health (1992a). *Effects of tobacco advertising on tobacco consumption: a discussion document reviewing the evidence*. Department of Health, London.

Department of Health (1992b). *The health of the nation. A strategy for health in England*. HMSO, London.

Department of Health (1993). *One year on . . . A report on the progress of the health of the nation*. Department of Health, London.

Department of Health (1994). *Smoke-free for health: an action plan to achieve the health of the nation targets on smoking*. Department of Health, London.

DHSS (Department of Health and Social Security) (1985). *Snuff-dipping—'Skoal Bandits'*. Letter from Chief Medical Officer, CMO (85) 6.

DHSS (Department of Health and Social Security) (1988). *Public health in England*. Report of the Committee of Inquiry into the future development of the public health function (Chairman Sir Donald Acheson). HMSO, London.

Donnan, P., Platt, S., Watson, J., Tannahill, A., and Raymond, M. (1994). Predictors of successful quitting: findings from a six-month evaluation of the *Smokeline* campaign. *Journal of Smoking-Related Disorders*, **5** (Suppl. 1), 271–6.

Downie, R. S. and Calman, K. C. (1994). *Healthy respect: ethics and health care*, (2nd edn). Oxford University Press.

Downie, R. S. and Fyfe, C. (1990). Health education in schools. In *Ethics in health education*, (ed. S. Doxiadis). Wiley, Chichester.

Downie, R. S. and Telfer, E. (1980). *Caring and curing*. Methuen, London.

Draper, P., Griffiths, J., Dennis, J., and Popay, J. (1980). Three types of health education. *British Medical Journal*, **281**, 493–5.

Everly, G. S., Smith, K. J., and Haight, G. T. (1987). Evaluating health promotion programmes in the workplace: behavioural models versus financial models. *Health Education Research*, **2**, 61–7.

Ewles, L. and Simnett, I. (1985). *Promoting health. A practical guide to health education*. Wiley, Chichester.

Ewles, L. and Simnett, I. (1992). *Promoting health: a practical guide*, (2nd edn). Scutari, London.

Family Heart Study Group (1994). Randomised controlled trial evaluating cardiovascular screening and intervention in general practice: principal results of British family heart study. *British Medical Journal*, **308**, 313–20.

FCM (Faculty of Community Medicine) (1988). *Alcohol. The prevention of problems related to its use*. FCM, London.

Festinger, L. (1957). *A theory of cognitive dissonance*. Stanford University Press.

Festinger, L. and Carlsmith, J. M. (1959). Cognitive consequences of forced compliance. *Journal of Abnormal and Social Psychology*, **58**, 203–10.

Frey, D. (1986). Recent research on selective exposure to information. In *Advances in experimental social psychology*, Vol. 19, (ed. L. Berkowitz). Academic Press, Orlando.

Fullard, E., Fowler, G., and Gray, M. (1987). Promoting prevention in primary care: controlled trial of low technology, low cost approach. *British Medical Journal*, **294**, 1080–2.

Gochman, D. S. and Saucier, J. F. (1982). Perceived vulnerability in children and adolescents. *Health Education Quarterly*, **9**, 142–55.

Goldberg, D. P. (1978). *Manual of the General Health Questionnaire*. NFER-Nelson, Windsor.

Green, L. W. (1977). Evaluation and measurement: some dilemmas for health education. *American Journal of Public Health*, **67**, 155–61.

Green, L. W. and Lewis, F. M. (1987). Data analysis in the evaluation of health education: toward standardization of procedures and terminology. *Health Education Research*, **2**, 215–21.

Green, L. W., Kreuter, M. W., Deeds, S. G., and Partridge, K. B. (1980). *Health education planning: a diagnostic approach*. Mayfield, Palo Alto.

Harrison, D. F. N. (1986). Editorial. Dangers of snuff, both 'wet' and 'dry'. *British Medical Journal*, **293**, 405–6.

Health Education Board for Scotland (1993). *Strategic plan 1992 to 1997*. Health Education Board for Scotland, Edinburgh.

Health Education Studies Unit (1982). *Final report of the patient project*. Health Education Council, London.

Health Promotion Authority for Wales (1990). *Health for all in Wales: strategies for action*. Health Promotion Authority for Wales, Cardiff.

Heider, F. (1944). Social perception and phenomenal causality. *Psychological Review*, **51**, 358–74.

Heider, F. (1958). *The psychology of interpersonal relations*. Wiley, New York.

Henerson, M. E., Morris, L. L., and Fitz-Gibbon, C. T. (1990). *How to measure attitudes*. Sage, Newbury Park.

Hovland, C. I. and Janis, I. L. (ed.) (1959). *Personality and persuasibility*. Yale University Press.

Hunt, S. M., McEwen, J., and McKenna, S. P. (1986). *Measuring health status*. Croom Helm, London.

ICRF (Imperial Cancer Research Fund) OXCHECK Study Group

(1994). Effectiveness of health checks conducted by nurses in primary care: results of the OXCHECK study after one year. *British Medical Journal*, **308**, 308–12.

ICRF OXCHECK Study Group (1995). Effectiveness of health checks conducted by nurses in primary care: final results of the OXCHECK study. *British Medical Journal*, **310**, 1099–104.

Illich, I. (1977). *Limits to medicine*. Penguin, Harmondsworth.

Kant, I. (1782). *Groundwork of the metaphysics of morals*, (1st edn) (ed. H. J. Paton) (1948). Hutchinson, London.

Kelly, M. P. (1989). Some problems in health promotion research. *Health Promotion*, **4**, 317–30.

Kelly, M. P. (1992). Health promotion in primary care: taking account of the patient's point of view. *Journal of Advanced Nursing*, **17**, 1291–6.

Kelly, M. P. and Charlton, B. G. (1992). Editorial. Health promotion: time for a new philosophy? *British Journal of General Practice*, **42**, 223–4.

Kelly, M. P. and Sullivan, F. (1992). The productive use of threat in primary care: behavioural responses to health promotion. *Family Practice*, **9**, 476–80.

Kendell, R. E., de Roumanie, M., and Ritson, E. B. (1983). Influence of an increase in excise duty on alcohol consumption and its adverse effects. *British Medical Journal*, **293**, 405–6.

King Edward's Hospital Fund for London (1989). *Blood cholesterol measurement in the prevention of coronary heart disease*. Consensus statement. King's Fund Centre, London.

Last, J. M. (ed.) (1988). *A dictionary of epidemiology*, (2nd edn). Oxford University Press.

Lawrence, D. (1981). The development of a self-esteem questionnaire. *British Journal of Educational Psychology*, **51**, 245–51.

Lazarus, R. (1976). *Patterns of adjustment*, (3rd edn). McGraw Hill, New York.

Lazarus, R. and Folkman, S. (1984). Coping and adaptation. In *Handbook of behavioural medicine*, (ed. W. Gentry). Guildford, New York.

Ley, P., Whitworth, M. A., Skilbeck, C. E., Woodward, R., Pinsent, R. J., Pike, L. A., Clarkson, M. E., and Clark, P. B. (1976). Improving doctor–patient communication in general practice. *Journal of the Royal College of General Practitioners*, **26**, 720–4.

Likert, R. (1932). A technique for the measurement of attitudes. *Archives of Psychology*, **140**, 44–53.

Maccoby, N. and Alexander, J. (1980). Use of media in lifestyle programmes. In *Behavioural medicine: changing health lifestyles*, (ed. P. O. Davidson and S. M. Davidson). Brunner Mazel, New York.

Maccoby, N. and Farquhar, J. W. (1975). Communication for health: unselling heart disease. *Journal of Communication*, **25**, 114–26.

McKeown, T. (1976). *The role of medicine: dream, mirage or nemesis?*, p. 108. Nuffield Provincial Hospitals Trust, London.

Marsh, A. and McKay, S. (1994). *Poor smokers*. No. 771 in Policy Studies Institute Research Report Series. Policy Studies Institute, London.

Medrich, E. A. (1979). Constant television: a background to daily life. *Journal of Communication*, **29**, 171–6.

Mencken, H. L. (1923). *Prejudices: third series*. Jonathan Cape, London.

Mill, J. S. (1859). *On liberty*, (ed. M. Warnock) (1962). Collins, London.

Mill, J. S. (1861). *Utilitarianism*, (ed. M. Warnock) (1962). Collins, London.

NALGO (National Association of Local Government Officers) (1984). *Health promotion and the grading of health education officers*. NALGO NHS Circular HS 6020, London.

NIDHSS (Northern Ireland Department of Health and Social Services) (1991). *A regional strategy for the Northern Ireland health and personal social services 1992–1997*. NIDHSS, Belfast.

Nutbeam, D. (1986). Health promotion glossary. *Health Promotion*, **1**, 113–27.

Nutbeam, D., Smith, C., and Catford, J. (1990). Evaluation in health education: A review of progress, possibilities, and problems. *Journal of Epidemiology and Community Health*, **44**, 83–9.

OPCS (Office of Population Censuses and Surveys) (1983). *Smoking attitudes and behaviour*. HMSO, London.

Osgood, C. E., Suci, G. J., and Tannenbaum, P. H. (1957). *The measurement of meaning*. University of Illinois Press.

Peters, R. S. (1973). *The philosophy of education*. Oxford University Press.

Pinet, G. (1987). Health legislation, prevention and ethics. In *Ethical dilemmas in health promotion*, (ed. S. Doxiadis). Wiley, Chichester.

Quigley, P. A. (1981). Prevention and health: no body's business. *Public Health* (London), **95**, 97–9.

Ribeaux, S. and Poppleton, S. E. (1978). *Psychology and work—an introduction*. Macmillan, London.

Roberts, J. L. (1986). *Code busting by tobacco companies*. North Western Regional Health Authority, Manchester.

Roberts, J. L. (1987). *More honour'd in the breach . . . how the 1986 voluntary agreement on tobacco advertising is being broken*. Project Smoke Free, Manchester.

Roediger, H. L., Rushton, J. P., Capaldi, E. D., and Paris, S. G. (1984). *Psychology*. Little, Brown, Boston.

Rosenberg, M. (1965). *Society and the adolescent self image*. Princeton University Press.

Russell, M. A. H., Wilson, C., Taylor, C., and Baker, C. D. (1979). Effect of general practitioners' advice against smoking. *British Medical Journal*, **2**, 231–5.

St Leger, A. S., Schnieden, H., and Walsworth-Bell, J. P. (1992). *Evaluating health services' effectiveness*. Open University Press, Milton Keynes.

Schools Council (1977*a*). *All about me 5–8*. Nelson, London.

Schools Council (1977*b*). *Think well 9–13*. Nelson, London.

Schools Council (1982). *Health education 13–18*. Forbes, London.

Scottish Office (1992). *Scotland's health: a challenge to us all*. HMSO, Edinburgh.

SHEG (Scottish Health Education Group) and SCCC (Scottish Consultative Council on the Curriculum) (1990). *Promoting good health: proposals for action in schools*. SHEG, Edinburgh.

Shickle, D. and Chadwick, R. (1994). The ethics of screening: is 'screeningitis' an incurable disease? *Journal of Medical Ethics*, **20**, 12–18.

Skrabanek, P. (1990). Why is preventive medicine exempt from ethical constraints? *Journal of Medical Ethics*, **16**, 187–90.

Smith, A. (1987). Qualms about QALYs. *Lancet*, **1**, 1134–6.

Smith, E. A. (1979). In *Health education. Perspectives and choices* (ed. I. Sutherland), p. 93. George Allen and Unwin, London.

SOHHD (The Scottish Office Home and health Department) (1991). *Health education in Scotland: a national policy statement*. The Scottish Office, Edinburgh.

Stone, D. and Stewart, S. (1994). *Towards a screening strategy for Scotland*. Scottish Forum for Public Health Medicine, Glasgow.

Tannahill, A. (1985*a*). Reclassifying prevention. *Public Health* (London), **99**, 364–6.

Tannahill, A. (1985*b*). What is health promotion? *Health Education Journal*, **44**, 167–8.

Tannahill, A. (1988*a*). Health for all by the year 2000. Promoting health in East Anglia. In *Promoting health in East Anglia*, Conference report. East Anglian Regional Health Authority, Cambridge.

Tannahill, A. (1988*b*). Editorial. *Community Medicine*, **10**, 94–7.

Tannahill, A. (1990). Health education and health promotion: planning for the 1990s. *Health Education Journal*, **49**, 194–8.

Tannahill, A. (1992). Epidemiology and health promotion: a common understanding. In *Health promotion: disciplines and diversity*, (ed. R. Bunton and G. Macdonald). Routledge, London.

Tannahill, A. (1994). *Health education and health promotion: from priorities to programmes*. No. 1 in World Health Organization Regional Office for Europe Health Promotion Country Series. Health Education Board for Scotland/World Health Organization, Edinburgh.

Tannahill, A. and Robertson, G. (1986). Health education in medical education: collaboration, not competition. *Medical Teacher*, **8**, 165–70.

Taylor, P. (1985). *The smoke ring: tobacco, money and multinational politics*. Sphere, London.

Thurstone, L. L. (1928). Attitudes can be measured. *American Journal of Sociology*, **33**, 529–54.

Tones, B. K. (1977). *Effectiveness and efficiency in health education: a review of theory and practice*. Scottish Health Education Unit, Edinburgh.

Tones, B. K. (1979). Past achievement and future success. Chapter 12 in *Health education: perspectives and choices*. George Allen and Unwin, London.

Tones, B. K. (1981). Affective education and health. In *Health education in schools*, (ed. J. Cowley, K. David, and T. Williams). Harper and Row, London.

Tones, B. K. (1983). Education and health promotion: new direction. *Journal of the Institute of Health Education*, **21**, 121–31.

Tones, B. K. and Tilford, S. (1994). *Health education: effectiveness, efficiency and equity*, (2nd edn). Chapman and Hall, London.

USNIH (United States National Institute of Health) (1986). *Health implications of smokeless tobacco*. Consensus development conference statement, Vol. 6, No. 1. NIH, Washington.

Vincent, A. and Plant, R. (1984). *Philosophy, politics and citizenship*. Blackwell, Oxford.

Wallston, K. A. and Wallston, B. S. (1978). Development of the Multidimensional Health Locus of Control (MHLC) scales. *Health Education Monographs*, **6** (2).

Walster, E. and Festinger, L. (1962). The effectiveness of 'overheard' persuasive communications. *Journal of Abnormal and Social Psychology*, **65**, 395–402.

Wheldall, K. (1975). *Social behaviour*. Methuen, London.

Whitehead, M. (1987). *The health divide: inequalities in health in the 1980s*. Health Education Council, London.

WHO (World Health Organization) (1946). *Constitution*. WHO, New York.

WHO (World Health Organization) (1984). *Health promotion. A discussion document on the concept and principles*. WHO, Copenhagen.

WHO (World Health Organization) (1985). *Targets for health for all*. WHO, Copenhagen.

WHO (World Health Organization) (1986). *Ottawa Charter for Health Promotion*. WHO, Geneva.

WHO (World Health Organization) (1991). *Health for all targets. The health policy for Europe*, (updated edition). WHO, Copenhagen.

WHO (World Health Organization), Council of Europe, and Commission of the European Communities (1993). *The European network of health promoting schools*. WHO, Copenhagen.

Williams, A. (1983). The economic role of 'health indicators'. In *Measuring the social benefits of medicine*, (ed. G. Teeling Smith). OHE, London.

Williams, G. (1984). Health promotion—caring concern or slick salesmanship? *Journal of Medical Ethics*, **10**, 191–5.

Williams, T. (1987). Health education in secondary schools. In *Health education in schools*, (ed. K. David and T. Williams). Harper and Row, London.

Wilson, J. M. G. and Jungner, G. (1968). *Principles and practice of screening for disease*. World Health Organization, Geneva.

Winn, D. M., Blot, W. J., Shy, C. M., Pickle, L. W., Toledo, A., and Fraumeni, J. F., Jr. (1981). Snuff dipping and oral cancer among women in the Southern United States. *New England Journal of Medicine*, **304**, 745–9.

Zajonc, R. B. (1968). Attitudinal effects of mere exposure. *Journal of Personality and Social Psychology, Monograph Supplement*, **9** (2), 1–27.

Index